BE YOUNG

The Ultimate Anti-Aging Guide to Maintaining Your Youth

BE YOUNG

The Ultimate Anti-Aging Guide to Maintaining Your Youth

By

Dr. Barry Dinner MD, MBBCH, ABAARM

First Edition 2018

ISBN 13: 978-1-7328884-2-5 (paperback)

LCCN Imprint Name: Beyoung Health INC
Number 2018912319

Printed in Israel

Published by Beyoung Health INC
Baltimore, Maryland

Visit: beyoung.life
Email: info@beyoung.life

AUTHOR'S CONTACT INFORMATION

Dr. Barry Dinner, MBBCH, ABAARM

Beyoung Health Inc.
410-943-7085
info@beyoung.life

Stay informed about the latest Anti-Aging developments, supplements and products. Subscribe to Dr. Barry Dinner's monthly newsletter, *Ignite Your Youth*, which provides practical advice on how you can truly "add life to your years" as well as "years to your life," along with the Complete Ignite Anti-Aging system and Dr. Dinner's LIFE Protocol.

Go to www.beyoung.life and subscribe now!

DISCLAIMER

The materials and content contained in this book are for general information and education purposes only and are not intended to be a substitute for professional medical advice, diagnosis or treatment. None of the information in this book should ever be interpreted as a claim of treatment or cure of any medical condition.

Readers of this book should not rely exclusively on information provided in this book for their own health needs. All specific medical questions should be presented to your own health care provider. Diagnosis and treatment of any medical conditions are strictly for you to discuss with your doctor.

The intention of this book is to provide information about anti-aging.

We also have attempted to provide anti-aging guidelines for maintaining your youth. None of the information in this book, and none of the guidelines should ever be interpreted as claims of diagnosis, treatment, or cure of any medical condition.

Beyoung Health Inc. and Dr. Barry Dinner do not assume any risk for your use of this book. In consideration for your use of this book, you agree that in no event will Beyoung Health Inc. and Dr. Barry Dinner be liable to you in any manner whatsoever for any decision made or action or non-action taken by you in reliance upon the information provided through this book.

All the information in this book is published in good faith and for general information purposes only. We do not make any warranties about the completeness, reliability and accuracy of this information, nor is anything in this book to be considered a guarantee of benefit or a claim of improvement for any medical condition. Any action you take upon the information on our website is strictly at your own risk, and we will not be liable for any losses and damages in connection with the use of the information in this book.

TABLE OF CONTENTS

ABOUT THE AUTHOR   xi

ACKNOWLEDGEMENTS   xiii

FOREWORD   1

INTRODUCTION   5

THE LIFE PROTOCOL   8

CHAPTER 1   19

Maintaining Cellular Health   19

CHAPTER 2   23

Lifestyle Factors   23

    2.1 Exercise   23

    2.2 Nutrition   35

    2.3 Stress and Adrenal Fatigue   44

    2.4 Attitude   51

    2.5 Sleep   53

CHAPTER 3   58

Purpose and Social Contact   58

CHAPTER 4   61

The Immune System   61

    4.1 Inflammation   63

    4.2 Cancer Prevention   67

CHAPTER 5   71

The Functional Systems   71

    5.1 The Cardiovascular System   71

    5.2 The Supply Lines — The Circulatory System   75

    5.3 The G.I. System   83

    5.4 The Liver   87

    5.5 The Brain and Nervous System   93

    5.6 The Kidney or Renal System   99

    5.7 The Musculoskeletal System   104

    5.8 Summary: Maintaining Strong Organ Systems   110

CHAPTER 6   114

The Endocrine System   114

    6.1 Thyroid   115

    6.2 Adrenal Hormones   117

    6.3 Pancreas   120

    6.4 Sex Hormones   122

CHAPTER 7   131

An Overview of How the Life Protocol Works Together   131

CHAPTER 8   136

Supplements for Each System and each Pathway to Slow
Aging   136

CHAPTER 9   143

Attitude: Aging, The Beginning of a New Life   143

CHAPTER 10   145

Break Limitations and Boundaries   145

CHAPTER 11   147

Beyoung's Program in a Nutshell   147

APPENDIX   151

GLOSSARY   164

ABOUT THE AUTHOR

Dr. Barry Dinner is a highly respected anti-aging physician, whose integrative approach to life extension has enabled him to imbue a healthy and meaningful quality of life into all those who seek his counsel. Dr. Dinner's anti-aging LIFE Protocol is predicated on three pillars — Lifespan, Youthspan and Valuespan — which have rekindled the youth of patients around the world.

Having graduated from the highly esteemed South African University of Witwatersrand's (WITS) Medical School with a bachelor's degree of Medicine and Surgery, Dr. Dinner's career spans more than thirty-three years, in which he developed sophisticated and advanced pro-active programs for preventive medicine in family practices, as well as serving as medical director for a 500-bed geriatrics hospital. Moreover, Dr. Dinner founded the highly successful Corporate Stress Institute of SA, having partnered with acclaimed psychology professors at the WITS School of Business in order to devise a program which combined both stress and health management.

After having practiced a wide range of medical disciplines, such as internal medicine, psychiatry, pediatrics, dermatology, obstetrics and gynecology, Dr. Dinner completed his fellowship in anti-aging and regenerative medicine with the American Academy of Anti-Aging Medicine in 2010.

Today, Dr. Dinner is active as an anti-aging practitioner and is the author of *Heart of the Matter.* He is the founder of Ignite Your Youth anti-aging nutritional supplements, an out-branch of his anti-aging clinic for advanced testing, cardiovascular health, brain health, bioidentical hormone replacement therapy, the management of metabolic illnesses, nutritional and fitness programs, as well as stress and adrenal fatigue management.

ACKNOWLEDGEMENTS

I would like to thank my amazing teachers in the field of anti-aging and functional medicine. This includes the professors and lecturers at A4M — The American Academy of Anti-Aging Medicine. I would like to make special mention of Dr. Pam Smith, the director and driver of the excellent programs; the fellowship in anti-aging medicine, Dr. Mark Houston, who has changed our understanding of vascular health; and Dr. James Lavelle, who engendered an unbelievable understanding of chemistry, pharmacology and the metabolic processes.

I would also like to thank Dr. Andrew Heiman, who provided a unique understanding of the various metabolic processes of the body; Dr Jill Carnahan, who through her own personal journey has become an expert in gastrointestinal and immune health; as well as Dr. Mark Rosenberg, who runs the unique integrative cancer treatment program.

During the course of my studies in anti-aging, I have gained a great deal of knowledge from the writings of Dr. Dale Bredersen, who has brought new hope to millions of Alzheimer's and potential Alzheimer's sufferers.

The unique common quality of these teachers and healers is their brilliance in being brave enough to forge into new territories in medicine and maintain the integrity of scientific process and accuracy.

A special thanks goes to Sahar Swidan, who is not only a brilliant pharmacist, but someone who can make up a remedy for almost any ailment. Not only have I gained extensive knowledge from her in the field of pharmacology and natural supplements, but she has advised and helped us with the compilation of all our formulas that we recommend.

I would like to thank Naomi Chait for her meticulous editing, research and help in completing my books and articles.

I would like to thank Barzillai for his constant support and invaluable input in the design of our formulas and of the program as a whole.

To my son Tsvi, I appreciate your tireless work and thoroughness in assuring all our programs and work processes are in place, and to my daughter Malka Berman, thank you for your research in all areas of our program.

Finally, to my partner in life, my wife Cherie, thank you for making everything possible for me.

FOREWORD

I am honored to be writing this forward for Dr. Barry Dinner's book *Be Young*, which is a great addition to our Personalized Medicine educational mission.

I am privileged to have known Dr. Dinner for a while now, from the time he was a student in our fellowship program on Personalized Medicine. His never-ending quest to continue to learn, to treat his patients and educate his colleagues in the field of personalized medicine, is relentless.

As we all age and read daily about the skyrocketing statistics of chronic disease and how we are failing in our mission to curb these illnesses, the timing of this book is impeccable. We need to learn new tools, to think outside of the box and really look at whole system physiology and optimization in order to ward off chronic disease and the exponential incidence of cancer.

The body works harmoniously as a symphony, but when one system is out of tune and is not functioning efficiently, the rest of the body will not function well. Therefore, this book does an amazing job of looking at root-cause medicine and disease while addressing, most importantly, cellular energy and health. As we all know, if you are not optimal, healthy, and energetic at the cellular level — which is your foundation — organs and systems will have a hard time functioning properly and at ideal levels.

1

All of us are looking for the magic pill and the fountain of youth. I love Dr. Dinner's educational mission to increase Lifespan, Youthspan and Valuespan by providing some of the tools necessary to achieve this goal. It is important to note, that yes, we all would like to live much longer, but it must have Valuespan. We believe personalized medicine is an additional weapon to address symptoms and disease that we cannot diagnose in traditional medicine and to help patients maintain memory, mobility, and function as they age.

As you read this book and embark on your own lifespan journey, I encourage you to implement the LIFE Protocol, which is laid out logically and in an easy-to-follow format for providers and patients who wish to gain more knowledge in this space.

Many studies have shown that lifestyle factors are important in influencing disease and are critical to implement for optimal function, such as clean and lean diets, intermittent fasting, exercise and sleep. When I teach now, I always say that we have one medical specialty, it is called INFLAMMATOLOGY, as many chronic diseases are linked to immune system dysfunction and inflammation. Therefore, addressing the immune system and inflammation is paramount to optimal health and for proper organ system function. The endocrine system and hormones are also critical not only for fertility and wellbeing, but act as cellular messengers with hundreds of other functions in the body collectively.

Forward

I thoroughly enjoyed reading this book, as I am sure you will too, together with expanding your knowledge in this field.

To Health, Wealth, and Happiness!

Sahar Swidan, Pharm.D., BCPS, ABAAHP, FAARFM, FACA

Be Young

INTRODUCTION

I have spent many years in family practice treating thousands of patients. As a physician, one of the most satisfying accomplishments is to make an accurate diagnosis and prescribe the cure. One feels useful and helpful. However, I always felt somewhat limited in my ability to treat many conditions. People would recurrently complain of weakness, fatigue, headaches and weight gain, amongst other symptoms. After many panels of tests and specialists, often no cause would be found and a vague diagnosis would have to be selected, like viral illness, chronic fatigue or stress.

A number of years ago, I decided to do a fellowship in anti-aging medicine at the American Academy of Anti-Aging, which is run by outstanding physicians and healthcare providers. From there, an exciting world opened up for me, and the great new science of anti-aging medicine, based on functional medicine, has become an integral part of my practice.

There are many diseases that afflict the elderly, including dementia and Alzheimer's disease. Through my anti-aging studies, I have learned what contributes to damage in the brain and the causation of this disease. Ongoing research in this field helps us continue to discover new anti-aging techniques and procedures and keeps us abreast of the latest discoveries.

I have learned how to assess metabolic processes by going back to basic medical science, and through this, solutions to many illnesses can be found. Learning about the hormone pathways again provided a method to replace and balance hormones in a safe and healthy way. Relearning how the body produces energy and techniques to enhance this process, as well as the significance of maintaining a healthy gut and its effect on different processes in the body, enabled me to turn my focus to finding root causes to various ailments.

I have seen over the years how so-called conventional medicine eventually comes to recognize the truth and the value of functional medicine, eventually incorporating these principles into practice. However, anti-aging and functional medicine principles remain ahead of the game in many areas.

Discovering the ultimate secret to maintaining our youth has been an ongoing search for hundreds of years. Many varieties of creams, lotions, vitamins and potions have been touted as the paramount solution to aging. However, the real question still remains, what is our understanding of the aging process in order to realistically slow it down. There is a tremendous amount of research being done in the anti-aging realm, both in the medical and functional fields and major progress has been achieved, but how much of it is practical and usable?

Introduction

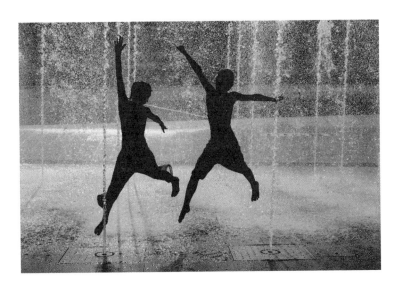

THE LIFE PROTOCOL

In recent years, vitamin and skin care companies have claimed that various supplements and natural products can make a difference in how you look and how you feel, and even conventional drug companies are now jumping on the bandwagon trying to claim their space in this field. It is therefore essential for the consumer to become well-informed on what really works and which interventions are useful. We are all consumers in this area, as we would all like to live longer and healthier lives. At my anti-aging clinic, we have analyzed many anti-aging techniques and hereby present a program with interventions that are worthwhile and that work.

Aging does not merely entail developing wrinkles and moving at a slower pace. It is a process which, over time, has multiple effects on all systems in our bodies, and if we understand the essential changes that occur with aging, we can then start addressing these root causes.

The change really occurs at the cellular level, meaning that every cell in the body ages. Inside each cell are mitochondria. They are small organelles that produce energy from oxygen metabolism. As we get older, these energy factories become fewer in number and less efficient, thereby affecting the functioning and structure of the systems of the body. For example, when a dysfunction of mitochondria occurs in the brain, Alzheimer's disease is usually the result.

When it occurs in the skin, it leads to a loss of elasticity, and in the bone, osteoporosis will develop.

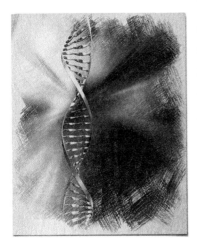

This same phenomenon will occur in all tissue and organs of the body. It is our priority to ensure that less damage occurs to the mitochondria, and that more growth factors exist to curb the aging and destruction of cells.

Besides the mitochondria, cells also contain the DNA for the replication of new cells and the genetic material that makes us who we are. At the end of each DNA strand is a cap called a telomere that protects the chromosomes, much like the plastic cap at the end of a shoelace. Without this cap, the lace becomes frayed and useless. With each cell division, the telomere shortens until it becomes too small for ongoing cellular division, and eventually leads to the death of the cell. An enzyme called telomerase ensures that the telomere remains at an adequate length, and it is important to make sure that the telomerase remains active and functioning.

Therefore, an essential part of anti-aging is ensuring that the correct factors are in place to preserve telomere length, thereby establishing and maintaining healthy DNA function. Negative factors that accelerate damage and destruction of our cells should be avoided. Whilst we are providing this healthful nourishment for the cells, we must take careful steps to prevent any elements that can encourage abnormal and uncontrolled cellular division, which leads to cancer.

My approach is to reinforce the maintenance of youthful healthy cells and in no way trigger abnormal DNA multiplication. Factors like antioxidants, certain minerals, vitamins, natural foods, natural anti-inflammatories and herbs have been proven to improve cellular health, whereas poor oxygenation of tissue, poor food choices and toxins have been shown to damage cells. This will be discussed in more detail later in the book.

Now it should be remembered that while there are many common factors that assist all organs and tissues, there are certain areas that have specific requirements. In our anti-aging program, we will not only provide a technique for cellular and mitochondrial health, but we also provide advice for specific organs and tissues.

Our approach to maintaining healthy organ function is to supply all the essential elements that the organ needs, and at the same time, encourage healthy utilization of that organ.

This would apply with the following systems:

The brain: We NEED TO work on enhancing the cells of the nervous system and improving the production and balance of the neurotransmitters that carry out many of the functions of the brain. This is done with the help of nutrient-rich brain food, and preventing toxins and destructive elements from reaching the brain cells. At the same time, we encourage the correct use of the brain to help maintain the brain tissue — for example, challenging your brain to learn a new language or study a new career.

The heart: We NEED TO provide the correct nutrients and coenzymes that help strengthen the heart muscle and improve the heart function. At the same time, we exercise the heart with different cardio exercises, which helps to keep it more efficient, fit and strong.

The vascular system: We NEED TO provide the correct minerals and nutrients to improve the blood vessels' inner lining (endothelium) and muscular layer. At the same time, we implement cardiovascular exercises to increase blood flow through the vessels.

The bones and muscle: We NEED TO provide essential vitamins and minerals that help build bone and muscle, as well as provide exercises to strengthen these tissues.

The main essence of our methodology is to provide the correct nutraceuticals for each system, whilst simultaneously building and strengthening them to maintain maximum functioning ability. This is consistent with the saying, "If you don't use it, you lose it." One of our most useful tools in our anti-aging program is to provide all the basic building blocks to support the organs and systems of the body, and then to use the body correctly and not abuse it. You cannot have one without the other.

It has now been proven beyond a doubt that many of the changes as a result of aging can be reversed. Although there is no magical anti-aging potion, reversing the effects of aging will not work without adjusting and optimizing your lifestyle. Conversely, there is no perfect lifestyle implementation without making sure you replace and replenish the minerals and nutrients that are essential for cellular functioning and removing harmful elements that are damaging. The LIFE Protocol is based on providing both of these solutions.

There are a number of theories and ideas that have been proposed about how to slow down the aging process, but many do not have enough evidence to prove they are correct. By reviewing all the theories that do work, the underlying theme of supplying the correct nutrients and keeping the mind and body active has a strong foundation that works.

My aim with the LIFE Protocol is to lengthen or enhance three parameters of one's life.

1. Lifespan
2. Youthspan
3. Valuespan

Lifespan
Our goal is to help increase the years of your life by using the best-known methods for life extension.

Youthspan
Our goal is to extend the youthful years as long as possible, so that even at a more

advanced age you can feel well and enjoy more youthful functionality. We hope to delay the onset of age-related illness.

Valuespan

Our goal is to help make the years that are gained useful and productive years, so that there will be personal growth and contribution with each and every day.

All the elements of the LIFE Protocol will contribute to extending the above spans. The LIFE Protocol will be divided into separate segments that together, will build your overall program. Each segment is interdependent, and it is important that the areas that have not been fully developed by you should be given extra attention and worked on. We have made the different areas very practical, so that once you have read the information, you can make real and lasting changes.

There are companies in the anti-aging arena that are presenting "hot off the press" interventions and products that seem to display anti-aging benefits. Proof may have been gleaned from a small human trial, or tests in animals or yeast, or other anecdotal information. Frequently, evidence comes to light that shows the converse, that in fact there is no benefit and sometimes even negative effects. This we have seen with the many fashions and fads that have entered the anti-aging space recently.

One example can be found in supplements containing NAD. NAD is an important coenzyme that is found in our cells and is involved with energy production. As we get older, the production of NAD slows down, which affects the functioning of the cells. Nicotinamide adenine dinucleotide (NAD+) can be replaced in a supplement and may have anti-aging benefits. However, studies have shown that NAD found in high levels is associated with an aggressive brain tumor called glioblastoma. We have to be sure that by enhancing cellular functioning we are not in fact stimulating cancer cells. I would therefore recommend waiting to assess whether NAD will enhance anti-aging without stimulating cancer, before taking it as an anti-aging supplement.

It is essential to have patience and wait and see which interventions in fact continue to advance and have staying power, and which develop negative side effects. We have made it our priority to wait sufficiently until we are satisfied that our choices display real and lasting benefits.

In presenting this program, I will indicate which nutraceuticals or interventions have strong evidence behind them and which may have less evidence. This will enable you to make choices which are likely to have the maximum benefit.

One needs a certain amount of honesty in this process, so that all ideas and suggestions are consistent with the best evidence available. However, if during the program a component is proven to be less than beneficial or even detrimental, it will be removed immediately from the protocol.

Motivation is a key factor in order to adopt and maintain an anti-aging protocol. The motivation must come from an understanding that it is worth making modifications in one's life that will alter the natural course of becoming old. Adopting a healthier lifestyle goes a long way in ensuring a longer life, with less chronic illness and less frailty in old age.

In order to get started, you have to place yourself in the right framework and set expectations for your anti-aging program. Ask yourself the following questions:

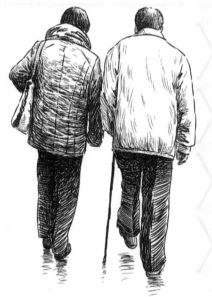

What do you want to be like at age 70?

Do you want to maintain your functionality as much as possible and be a healthy 70 year old?

Do you want to set your sights on being youthful at 70 and be in a physical condition to begin a new direction in life?

Would you like to be able to participate in serious exercise workouts a few times a week, or even become a major contributor to an organization that could use your skills?

In other words, you need to focus on achieving a beginning of a new life — rather than the beginning of the end of your old life.

Please remember that before embarking on an anti-aging program, you must do the basic age-related screening tests. If you have a family history or a personal history of a particular medical problem, then you should take this more seriously.

There are guidelines for breast, colon, prostate, skin and cervical cancer screening that can be discussed with your physician. Make sure that you are doing the best screening tests relative to your own family and personal history. It is obviously not going to be of any use to embark on an anti-aging program if you miss a preventable but potentially fatal disease, by not taking the time to discuss these screening tests with your physician.

All elements of the LIFE protocol are important. No two individuals are the same, however, each person has their own strengths and weaknesses and therefore will need to focus on certain areas more than others.

Gaining an understanding of your strengths and weaknesses, as well as which systems require boosting, is important to help you focus on your weaker areas. We have designed the Beyoung Quiz to help you identify the areas in your health which may cause you problems. This can be found on the Beyoung website at www.beyoung.life. This is a basic assessment, and of course, doing an in-depth anti-aging assessment with a qualified anti-aging physician, will provide a much more comprehensive understanding of what interventions are needed.

Our anti-aging program is not just about incorporating some vitamins and minerals into your diet, it is about a lifestyle change. It becomes a new way of life. A health and life program needs to be practical and easy to manage. The lifestyle changes must be straightforward to adopt and to maintain, and should even become enjoyable. Our LIFE protocol consists of the sections represented by L-I-F-E. Every section is important, and taken together, will make a tremendous positive impact on your health and longevity.

In the LIFE protocol, there are certain sections that have a global effect on the entire body down to the cellular level. These are the master influences and must be kept in top working order. They are universal and relevant to everyone's anti-aging program. One can compare these systems to the engine of the car, the power center that makes the car go. If one wire or spark plug doesn't work, the entire engine is faulty. The following factors influence all areas and functions of the body and are relevant to everyone:

- ❏ **Lifestyle factors**
- ❏ **Immune system and low inflammation**
- ❏ **Hormone balance**

There are also a number of requirements for the ideal functioning of all the main organs and systems of the body. These can be compared to the individual parts of the car. They may be more relevant to individuals who have weaknesses in a particular area and include:

- ❏ **Cardiovascular system**
- ❏ **Brain and nervous system**
- ❏ **Gastrointestinal system**
- ❏ **Musculoskeletal systems**
- ❏ **Liver and kidney**

As I described above, before we look at the specific systems of the body, we need to work on the core factors that cause aging — the main engine — which means maintaining cellular health.

CHAPTER 1

MAINTAINING CELLULAR HEALTH

Cellular health refers to the cells functioning well, communicating, reproducing, receiving ample nourishment, producing energy and performing the thousands of tasks that they are designed to do. However, we live in a toxic world where we are exposed to many chemicals, processed foods, excessive use of prescription drugs, high stress levels and the like, which can damage these vital cells and prevent them from performing properly.

There are different systems that supplement and nurture the cells throughout our body. Maintaining these systems and keeping them healthy, will have an overall effect on our health. The circulatory system, which is composed of capillaries and tiny blood vessels, supplies all the cells of the body with nutrients and oxygen and removes toxins and carbon dioxide. The nervous system reaches all cells and influences cell function via chemicals called neurotransmitters. The endocrine system sends hormones to different tissues and binds to receptors on the cell membrane that causes reactions in the cells. The immune system is made up of cells that search for foreign invaders such as viruses, bacteria and certain toxins, which help protect the cells and tissues from intruders.

19

Therefore, the master systems mentioned above must be kept in healthy working order. This includes healthy blood vessels, balanced hormones and well-functioning nervous and immune systems. These are the pillars of an anti-aging program and influence the basic functioning of all cells and organs of the body. Dysfunction of these systems leads to the breakdown of the body on the cellular level and causes accelerated aging.

When energy is produced from oxygen and glucose in the mitochondria of the cells, free radicals are created as a by-product, which can themselves damage the mitochondria. Taking adequate antioxidants, whether in the form of supplements or superfoods, will help counteract these free radicals. The following factors optimize cellular and mitochondrial health:

- ❏ Eating healthy nutrients
- ❏ Avoiding unhealthy foods
- ❏ Sufficient exercise
- ❏ Maintaining a good hormone balance (especially thyroid hormones, estrogen, progesterone, testosterone, maintaining low insulin and low cortisol levels — the stress hormone)
- ❏ Decreasing inflammation in the body
- ❏ Removing toxins from the body
- ❏ Taking the correct minerals and vitamins
- ❏ Taking adequate antioxidants

The details of this will be discussed in the following sections of the book and are indicated for general use for everyone.

The section on functional systems of the body relates to specific organ systems that need to be treated on a case-by-case basis, depending on one's own strengths and weaknesses.

The **LIFE** Protocol consists of the following sections:

LIFESTYLE FACTORS
- Exercise
- Nutrition
- Stress management
- Attitude
- Sleep

HEALTHY IMMUNE SYSTEM
- A strong immune system
- Reduced inflammation and autoimmune reactions
- Cancer prevention strategies

OPTIMIZING THE MAIN FUNCTIONAL SYSTEMS OF THE BODY
- The cardiovascular and circulatory system
- The gastrointestinal system
- The liver system
- The brain and nervous system
- The kidney and renal system
- The musculoskeletal system

THE ENDOCRINE SYSTEM

- The thyroid gland and thyroid hormones
- The adrenal hormones
- The pancreas and pancreatic hormones
- The sex hormones in males and females

CHAPTER 2

LIFESTYLE FACTORS

2.1 Exercise

There is nothing more beneficial and central to reversing aging than exercise. You can begin a routine at any age and you don't have to be an expert to start. Many aspects of poor health and indeed even illnesses can be reversed by increasing your fitness level. Keeping yourself in good shape is synonymous with heart strength, muscle strength and bone strength and can help improve metabolic problems, like diabetes, lipid problems and obesity. Exercising is also known to bump up the brain's feel-good neurotransmitters, called endorphins, which help reduce stress, and has been proven to prevent the onset of dementia.

There are three areas of fitness that are all equally important and should be included in a balanced program. They are aerobic fitness, flexibility and strength training. It is important to realize that as one gets older, muscle strengthening exercises become crucial, and more time must be spent on this.

Selecting a realistic and enjoyable exercise program will ensure that it is sustainable and not just a fleeting pastime. It is almost impossible to maintain a program that is difficult and unpleasant. Choosing an exercise routine that incorporates a variety of exercise types will help motivate you to keep working at it and will make exercising more enjoyable. If you are not already exercising, starting a routine can be quite daunting. Just remember, although it may take time to get used to working out, it should eventually become enjoyable.

The following categories of exercise should be built into your work-out program. Developing the right program for you is essential, as everyone has different needs and preferences. It is definitely not a case of one routine is good for everyone. The emphasis on the type of

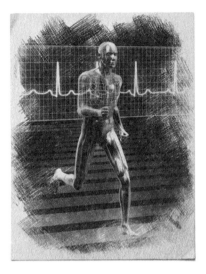

exercises will be influenced by your specific health profile and areas that need to be strengthened. Make sure that you do sufficient warm-up stretches before starting any exercise routine.

A. _Aerobics_

Aerobic exercise, which is also referred to as cardio, helps improve the efficiency of the heart and lungs by intensifying our breathing and heart rate. It results in increased fitness and improved physical and emotional health. Although cardio machines may be used when exercising, they are not necessary.

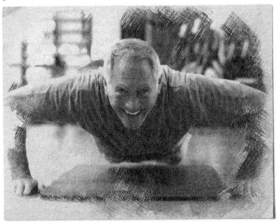

Aerobics exercises should be done for at least 30 minutes a day and can be broken up into three 10-minute workout sessions. The aim is to raise the heart rate to about 60-80% of the maximum heart rate. To calculate your maximum heart rate, take 220 less your age and times that by 60-80%. For example, if you are 50 years old, the formula would be 220-50=170 * 60%=102 beats per minute, and you can eventually increase it to 170 * 80%=136 beats per minute. You should be able to talk whilst exercising, but with difficulty. Examples of aerobic exercise are swimming, running, cycling, aerobic classes, dancing and skiing.

B. *Strength Training*

This intense type of exercising, also known as anaerobic training, builds power, strength and muscle. An example is weightlifting. The benefit of strength training is that it helps increase muscle mass and reduce fat tissue as well as build bone mass, which is extremely important in the prevention of osteoporosis.

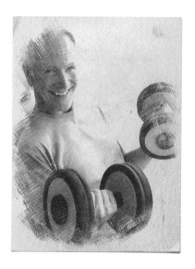

Muscle is a very active tissue that burns calories even when you sleep, whereas fat tissue is metabolically inactive and in fact, increases the body's inflammation and insulin resistance.

There are different muscle groups, all of which should be exercised to maintain your full strength; they include the peripheral muscles — the forearms, arms, shoulders, thighs and lower legs, and the core muscles — abdominal and back muscles, pelvic muscles and gluteus muscles. Gym circuits are well-equipped with different exercise equipment that strengthen the various muscle groups, and gym instructors are onsite to assist you with developing a strength training program.

It is quite useful and practical to buy some simple equipment, such as bands and dumbbells, to use at home.

You can create your own workout program to strengthen your muscles with the help of the internet or a gym instructor. Make sure you use exercise sites that are reliable and choose exercises that are sensible and applicable for you. The basis for a home workout routine should include a set of exercises for each muscle group, with 10 repetitions of each exercise to make up one set. As you build up your strength, you can increase this to 2 or 3 sets and increase the number of times you do the exercise or the repetitions.

Core exercises are very important building blocks but are often neglected. The area of your body referred to as the core is your midsection, including your abdomen, back and sides, and these muscles work as the stabilizers for the entire body. So, what is core training? Core exercises train the muscles in your pelvis, lower back, hips and abdomen to work in harmony. This leads to improved posture, stability and balance, whether during exercise or in daily activities. Strong core muscles can help you swing a golf club with ease, reach for a glass on the top shelf of your cupboard or bend down to tie your shoelace.

Nowadays, more jobs are technology based, which means sitting for long periods of time behind a computer. This weakens the core muscles. However, exchanging an exercise ball for a chair can maintain your balance, posture and strengthen your muscles at the same time. Additional fitness ball exercises, sit-ups, planks and bridge exercises should all be incorporated into your workout routine.

It is hard not to notice elderly people walking with their shoulders stooped, their backs rounded and their heads facing the ground. Although this seems a natural part of aging, it need not be the case. Strengthening your core muscles and maintaining an upright posture can prevent you from looking frail and hunched over. Make sure you sit upright at all times and do not slouch in your chair. Walk with your shoulders pulled back and your back and head upright and straight. Exercises can prevent and even reverse this unhealthy stance — for example, shoulder rolls, standing side slides and yoga.

C. *Flexibility*

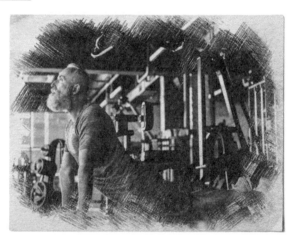

Flexibility training includes exercises that help increase the range of motion. The benefits include being able to perform better, especially in sports and daily tasks, with little risk of an injury. Remaining flexible helps preserve the range of movements in your joints, making everyday chores easy to do and enabling you to maintain functionality. Examples of flexibility training include both yoga and pilates classes, which focus on stress-relief, flexibility, strength, control, and endurance.

D. *Interval Training*

Interval training, which in years gone by was practiced solely by athletes, is a combination of short high-intensity activity followed by low-intensity recovery exercise. This is repeated a number of times during one exercise session. It is a great way to burn extra calories and stay in excellent shape. For example, if you enjoy speed walking, intersperse short bouts of jogging in between. This will enable you to burn more calories while decreasing your exercise time — instead of walking for 60 minutes, you can walk/run for 45 minutes.

There are a number of benefits to incorporating interval training into your daily routine: you can stave off boredom by integrating bursts of variety, no additional equipment is necessary, your fitness level will increase and you will burn extra calories. High intensity workouts help you build muscle and lose more fat. It is very beneficial for heart health to push yourself hard and to get your heart rate up and then to take small recovery periods in between.

Do not begin interval training without consulting your physician first, especially if you have a chronic illness. It is safe for most people to incorporate it into their normal exercise routine, however, start off slowly so that you do not damage any muscles, tendons or bones. Examples of incorporating interval training into your training routine are jogging interspersed with fast running; jumping rope at a high speed for 60 seconds followed by light jumping for 3 minutes; and running up a long flight of stairs as fast you can and then jogging down the stairs slowly. These high intensity and recovery phases should be repeated at least 7 times or until a good workout has been achieved.

E. *Non-Exercise Exercise, Daily Activities*

Technology today has made our lives easier, but at the same time, more sedentary. We spend a lot of time in front of the TV or computer at home or at work, we drive or use public transport instead of walking, shopping can be ordered at the click of a button and household chores have become far less demanding. If you work at a desk for long hours, ensure that you take sufficient breaks to walk around and stretch your muscles. Walk around the block during your lunch hour and try exchanging an exercise ball for your office chair in order to maintain muscle control and balance.

Devices like Fitbits, which monitor your steps, are helpful in reminding you to keep moving and to achieve a certain number of steps a day. Sitting the whole day may be one of the most dangerous occupations, making intermittent walking essential.

You should build an exercise program in a balanced fashion, so that strength exercises are done about 3 to 4 times a week, with breaks in between sessions to allow for muscle recovery. Individuals over the age of 50 years should incorporate muscle strengthening exercises into their routine to help maintain muscle strength, because muscle weakness is reversible at any age.

An aerobic exercise program needs to be included at least 3 times per week in order to maintain cardiovascular fitness. Anything less than this will not provide accumulative fitness, and any benefit gained with a few sessions can be lost quickly.

Interval training is an excellent solution for a quick way to achieve aerobic fitness and it also contributes to muscle strengthening. Studies show that interval training builds endurance and burns calories faster, as well as improves heart health.

It is important to remember that even if you have a good fitness program in place, it is essential to move a lot during the day. Sitting for long periods is not healthy and we encourage using devices like a Fitbit and the Beyoung tracker to remind you to move.

Flexibility is essential in order to prevent stiffness and muscle pains. We frequently attribute stiffness and pain to arthritis and joint problems, but it may be due to muscle stiffness and is reversible with stretching exercises.

F. *Balance Exercises*

The human gait pattern is defined as the way people walk and balance. This gait pattern is responsible for our ability to maintain an upright posture. Balance is the ability of the body to uphold an upright position and respond quickly to a situation that causes you to become unstable, such as walking on an uneven walking surface.

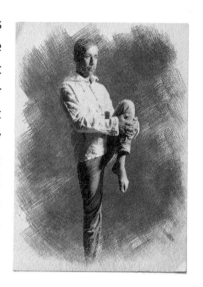

Balance exercises are good for people of all ages to practice. It prevents falls and builds self-confidence in older adults by helping them feel in control of their movements and not be afraid to go places and do things for fear of falling. There are over 2 million emergency room visits per year in America from elderly people who have fallen; many of them could have been prevented if balance exercises had been done. No equipment is necessary for balance exercises, which can be practiced anytime and anywhere. If need be, a chair can be placed nearby and used as a balancing crutch.

Remember, the above is only a brief outline of a good exercise program. For more in-depth information and examples of different exercises, look at exercise/health sites online. Alternatively, a fitness coach can instruct you on how to plan and implement a good home exercise plan, or you can join a gym and have access to a trainer and a wide variety of equipment.

I have a treadmill, dumbbells, an exercise mat and some bands at home, and my exercise routine is as follows:

1. I warm up and stretch and then do a set of strength exercises, covering all the muscle groups.
2. Then I do interval training on the treadmill and another set of strength exercises.
3. I repeat step 2 again and then cool down.

It takes me 30–40 minutes to do this routine and I cover all bases for fitness. In between this routine, I do a relaxed run or cycle one to two days a week.

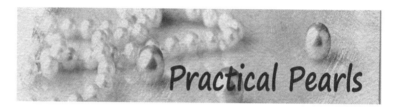

Practical Pearls

1. *Make exercise and movement a part of your life, and start enjoying the benefits of feeling stronger and fitter.*

2. *Stretch before each exercise session.*

3. *Do at least 3 sessions of muscle-strengthening exercises per week.*

4. *Do at least 3 sessions of aerobic exercises per week, including interval training.*

5. *Make sure you move a lot even when you are not exercising. Do not sit passively for extended periods. Housework is good physical work, and if done at a fast pace, it increases your heart rate and can count as part of your daily exercise.*

6. *Be conscious of your posture whilst standing, sitting and walking. Make sure you hold your head and shoulders back and sit straight and upright when in a chair.*

7. *Maintain your balance with the help of exercises.*

8. *Take 10 minutes to plan your program in the Beyoung health tracker, and then check off each time you do a session of exercise. This will motivate you to achieve your weekly plan.*

2.2 Nutrition

In this section, we will present the principles of good nutrition. It has now been proven that healthy nutrition has huge benefits for your overall health. It plays a major role in preventing heart disease, Alzheimer's, diabetes and many cancers. Autoimmune diseases, gastrointestinal diseases and many allergies can all be reduced through the correct diet. The details and practical application of a healthy eating program is provided with links to the appropriate sections on our internet site.

Maintaining a healthy diet comes with practice, but is within everyone's reach. Processed, ready-made foods are quick and easy to put in the microwave or oven, but lack nutrients and are packed with food coloring and additives. Meals need to be simple and enjoyable, with little preparation and fuss, but filled with nutrients and fresh ingredients. By changing the food items in your home and applying a few basic healthy principles, getting used to healthy eating habits should be relatively straightforward and easy.

Eating healthier meals is not the same as dieting, which pushes you into a mode of depriving yourself of food and getting little enjoyment from what you eat. If you do not have the willpower to stay on a diet, you end up cheating here and there and eventually succumb to the temptation of eating chocolates, junk food, burgers and Coke again. This leads to yo-yo dieting, where people are continuously starting a new diet and then breaking it, and although they are in a state of deprivation, they never lose weight or become healthy.

The alternative to dieting is to add good quality nutritious food to your repertoire of cooking. Emphasis is placed more on what you eat and not so much on the quantity. A positive attitude towards adopting a healthy diet will keep you on track and encourage you to make the necessary changes. Eating a certain way is habitual, and by omitting unhealthy foods from your shopping lists, you will not have these food items in your pantry and thus will be less tempted. Make sure you use whole grains and fresh ingredients, and aim to become healthy and not to become thin. You will automatically lose weight but not be hooked into the weight-loss success/failure model.

Beyoung Clinics has created an easy-to-use Healthy Living app to steer you in the right direction and help keep you on track with your diet. It helps you set specific eating goals for yourself and motivates you to remain on target. Besides tracking your eating habits for you, it also records your exercise and fitness routines.

The concept of the Beyoung nutrition app is that it is designed to encourage, direct and remind you to convert to healthy choices each day and each week, gradually helping you to eliminate unhealthy foods. The idea is not to watch calories or adhere to a specific diet, but rather to spell out what you should eat each day, with some foods being eaten a few times a week. The nutrition plan is based on a point system where you gain points eating healthy choices and lose points for unhealthy foods.

There are three categories of food: the green, yellow and red sections. Foods that should be eaten daily or weekly form the basis of your diet and are found in the green category.

The second category, or the yellow group, includes foods that should be eaten in moderation and used as add-ons to the green foods. An example would be a good fresh salad with a few pieces of organic chicken added. Or a delicious cooked vegetable stir-fry with a small amount of beef slices from grass-fed animals. The idea is to mainly eat the nutritious green area foods and have small amounts from the yellow category sprinkled in.

The third area or red area foods should be avoided, as they are unhealthy choices and contain ingredients that may contribute to many diseases that occur as we age. The idea of adhering to this app is that once you get used to this way of eating, it will become second nature, and the right foods will become your first choice.

An example of the three food categories is listed in the appendix.

Once you have made the important decision to change your eating habits, the next step is to prepare for your program.

Firstly, remove all the food items that are not healthy and that tempt you from your home or work area. We generally eat what is readily available and within our radar.

Remove all foods with a high sugar content. Items containing cane sugar — and especially high fructose corn syrup — should be not be in your pantry. Get into the habit of reading food labels and familiarize yourself with what is contained in different foods. Avoid buying sugary drinks, sodas and artificial fruit juices, which contain extra calories and promote obesity. Water, herbal teas and fresh fruit juices are a healthier alternative.

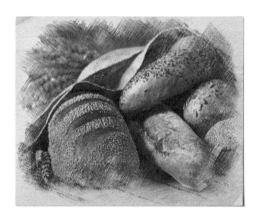

It is important to reduce refined carbohydrates in your diet, including products made from refined wheat such as cereals, bagels, pastries, white bread and pasta. White potatoes and white rice should also be kept to a minimum. Healthier alternatives include whole wheat breads, pastas and quinoa and baked foods made from spelt, oat, barley or the like.

Over the years, low fat, no-fat and high-fat diets have been an issue of contention, as differing fads have dictated the best diets for that particular season. Although the amount of fat in diets has differed, certain types are known to be detrimental to your health and should be avoided. These include trans fats, hydrogenated and partially hydrogenated fats, which are oils that have been processed and hydrogenated. They become solid like margarine and are used in many baked goods. Any food label with trans fats or partially hydrogenated oils included in the ingredients should be avoided. This is usually found in store-bought cookies, crackers, margarine, frozen pizza, fried fast foods and microwave popcorn.

Healthy fats and oils are good choices and have major health benefits. They are found in nuts, avocados, olive oil, coconut oil, and omega-3 oils from fish, all of which should be added to your diet. The best fish choices are represented by the abbreviation SMASH. Salmon (from cold water sources, not farmed), mackerel, anchovies, sardines and herring.

There are a number of other good protein sources besides fish which should be included in your diet. Meat obtained from grazed animals is the best option, as they are grass fed and do not eat unhealthy animal feed, nor are they fattened up with hormones. Poultry should be organic and free range as the normal store-bought chickens are usually pumped with hormones and antibiotics. Organic eggs should be used, as they have a high protein content. The final protein source is plant-based protein in the form of beans, legumes and quinoa.

The next step is to stock up your pantry with healthy foods. The fresher and less processed the ingredients, the better it is for you. Incorporating plenty of fresh fruit and vegetables into your diet provides you with minerals and vitamins with little fuss and effort. Choose foods that contain whole grains without hydrogenated oils, and try to avoid the junk food trap. Ensure you have plenty of good quality drinking water, which can be enjoyed with a slice of lemon for a refreshing taste. We have included a list of tips for healthy shopping in the appendix to help get you started.

Superfoods are a great addition to your diet and should be readily available to eat a few times a week. These include blueberries, avocados, green tea, broccoli, salmon, flaxseed, chia seeds, kale and pomegranates, to name a few.

Now that you know **what** to eat, we will discuss **how** to eat.

No Dieting

Diets are equivalent to self-denial and feeling hungry a lot of the time. They are often not sustainable for very long, and most people break them and then relapse to poor eating. As I have explained above, the essence of healthy eating is "replacement," which means removing poor food choices and replacing them with healthy choices. This change becomes enjoyable as one experiences the benefits of feeling good and losing weight. One acquires the taste of healthy foods and loses the desire for unhealthy choices. For example, sugar is an addiction, but the less one eats sugar the less one desires sugar. Conversely, the more one eats a healthy salad with nuts and a delicious healthy dressing, or a colorful, healthy stir-fry, the more one desires this type of food.

Eat Slowly, Enjoy Your Food

There are two types of people in the world. Those that eat to feel full, who get their satisfaction from a full feeling, and those that eat to enjoy the tastes and sensation of eating, who do not need to feel full. The first group of individuals eats rapidly in order to fill up and are always worried that there may not be enough for second helpings. They are obviously the heavier group. The second group eats slowly and savors the taste of the food, stopping to eat much sooner. They tend to be much lighter in weight.

It is essential to become a slow, mindful eater. You need to sit down when eating a meal, chew your food well, enjoy the tastes and place your fork down between each bite. This is mindful eating!

Don't get too hungry and don't get too full. The key is to create a balance, which is vital when it comes to nutrition. Not eating balanced meals at set times or skipping meals can result in extreme hunger and the desire to eat whatever you can put into your mouth first. This usually tends to be unhealthy foods and snacks, which can cause sugar highs and lows and a feeling of unsatisfied fullness. Eating because you are so hungry, can cause you to overeat and become overly full, which is unhealthy and unsatisfying.

It is important to drink enough fluids throughout the day. When we are hot during the summer months, we tend to get thirstier and drink more often. However, in winter it is easy to forget to drink because we don't have the same thirst. Make sure you keep well-hydrated with water or herbal teas.

Avoid sodas and sugar-filled fruit drinks, which add empty calories to your diet and do little to quench your thirst. It is also a good idea to have a glass or two of water before a meal to help decrease your capacity to overeat.

Eat an early dinner and try not to eat again until the morning. Research has shown that finishing your dinner at least three hours before going to bed helps keep your weight in check, reduces the bloated feeling when going to bed and decreases the chance of having reflux whilst you sleep. It is also very beneficial to have a 12-hour mini fast, from dinner until the morning. The body utilizes fat for energy during that time, which has multiple benefits. Snacking into the night is a bad habit and leads to an inability to lose weight. Try getting into a routine of not eating again after an early dinner!

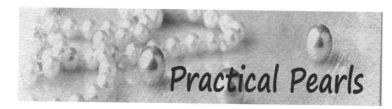

Practical Pearls

1. *Remove unhealthy food and snacks from your pantry and workplace.*

2. *It is OK to have an occasional treat without feeling guilty.*

3. *Sit down when you eat and eat slowly and mindfully. Put your fork down after each bite and chew your food well. This takes practice, especially in our fast-paced world where time is always of the essence.*

4. *Use vegetables as the basis for your meals. Make salads and stir fries either as a side dish or a main with a protein added.*

5. *It is good to spend time making tasty, healthy foods like delicious soups and well-spiced vegetables and salads.*

6. *Include superfoods in your diet a few times a week.*

7. *Record your meals in the Beyoung health tracker so that you become used to adding healthy choices and cutting back on unhealthy ones.*

8. *Remember, the healthier you eat, the less you will crave unhealthy foods.*

2.3 Stress and Adrenal Fatigue

The autonomic nervous system, which is comprised of two components, is a control system that acts subconsciously and modulates many automatic functions within the body, such as breathing, the heartbeat and various digestive processes. It has two separate branches, namely the sympathetic nervous system, which is stimulated in a "fight-or-flight" mode, and the parasympathetic system, which is known as the "rest-and-digest" mode. These systems seem to work in opposite ways, where one system encourages a physiological action and the other inhibits it.

When we need to defend ourselves from danger, the sympathetic nervous system jumps into action, driving blood from our digestive system to our skeletal muscles, dilating our pupils to help enhance our far vision and quickening our breathing to increase our oxygen intake. This system will also be turned on by the brain perceiving danger, such as when we are stressed. These reactions help us in the short term, such as during an intense period of danger, but if they are prolonged, they could lead to negative side effects that have an influence on our health.

When the body is working under the parasympathetic influence, all the systems are functioning in a safe mode. This is the rest-and-digest system — the heart rhythm is normal, food is easily digested and the stress hormones are at bay.

The vagus nerve is the main parasympathetic nerve which runs from the brain down to the abdomen. It is extremely important to ensure that the vagus nerve tone remains strong by keeping it stimulated and active. Productive activities, such as creative stimulation and healthy social contacts, are ways to achieve this. Additional techniques to eradicate stress and turn on vagal tone are described in my second book, *Heart of the Matter*.

Stress is one of the key players influencing health and longevity. When a person suffers chronic stress, despite having an excellent overall health profile, most of their health parameters will be negatively influenced. In fact, stress is a major cause of dementia, heart disease, high blood pressure, immune problems, gastrointestinal problems and many other illnesses.

The main focus is to live as much as possible in a relaxed, parasympathetic mode, with minimal stress levels.

When we are stressed for a prolonged period of time, our stress hormones are depleted and our body enters a state called adrenal fatigue or burnout. Adrenal fatigue is a syndrome resulting from the low functioning of the adrenal glands. The adrenal glands sit above the kidneys and are responsible for producing various hormones, including cortisol, aldosterone, adrenaline and noradrenaline. These hormones play a crucial role in maintaining metabolism, regulating salt and water balance in the body, as well as being responsible for the stress-related fight-or-flight response.

The brain has an inbuilt mechanism to produce or block the production of cortisol. Signals sent along the hypothalamic-pituitary-adrenal axis regulate the cortisol levels. Any slight change in the brain function as a result of too much stimulation, can cause either an over- or under-production of cortisol in the adrenal glands. Initially, with increased stress, the brain signals the adrenals to increase production of cortisol to deal with the stress. However, prolonged high cortisol levels will cause the brain to relay a message to stop producing cortisol, which leads to adrenal fatigue.

Symptoms of Adrenal Fatigue

There are common symptoms that people suffering from adrenal fatigue display, although not all the symptoms listed below are experienced by everyone. This in itself makes the illness complicated to diagnose. They are as follows:

- Extreme fatigue, mainly in the mornings and afternoons and a second wind at night
- Brain fog
- Food cravings for sweet or salty foods
- Memory disturbance
- Moodiness and irritability
- Depression
- Sleep disturbances
- Weight gain
- Inability to cope with even mildly stressful situations

Treatment of Adrenal Fatigue

1. One of the first lines of defense in treating adrenal fatigue is adhering to a nutritional diet plan and avoiding foods that aggravate the syndrome. When you are stressed,

healthy eating habits are usually ignored, meals are skipped and less nutritious food is consumed. Nutritional deficiencies put a strain on the adrenals and it is important to take vitamin supplements and eat a balanced diet to help counteract this. Vitamins help balance cortisol levels that affect the body's stress response and metabolism mechanism. There are some herbs and nutrients that are known to eliminate fatigue, by revitalizing the adrenal glands through balancing the hormones it produces.

2. As mentioned above, stress is the root cause of adrenal fatigue. Toxic relationships, whether at work or between family or friends, intensify emotional stress and need to be dealt with in order to help reduce adrenal fatigue. This might involve leaving a bad relationship, moving jobs or attending therapy sessions. It is essential to identify the source of the stress and be willing to deal with the issue. One may have to make major changes to remove the stress, but it will be worthwhile in the long run.

3. Getting a good, restful sleep each night is very important in repairing the adrenal glands and reducing stress levels. Between 10 p.m. and 1 a.m., the adrenals work the hardest to heal the body. When we push ourselves beyond 11 p.m. at night, the adrenal glands shift into high gear, giving us a "second wind" and putting strain on them. Therefore, going to bed before 11 p.m. and waking up after 8 a.m. is the most valuable sleep time an

individual can get, and even more so when suffering from adrenal fatigue.

4. In addition to working hard at reducing stressful conditions in your life, incorporating relaxation techniques into your daily routine can go a long way in helping to reduce stress. The main aim is to increase your vagal tone and make the vagus nerve the dominant influence on the body. We know that vagal tone is stimulated by doing worthwhile creative activities or participating in heartwarming social programs. In addition, certain practical techniques increase the vagus tone and relax the body; these include breathing exercises — which can be done anywhere, anytime — as well as meditation and guided imagery.

5. Exercise is an exceptional oxygenator and phenomenal stress reducer. If done correctly, exercise is a pivotal component to adrenal recovery. The key is to adjust the level of exercise according to one's capability, physical strength and overall health. However, it is important to remember that more is not necessarily better, as over-exercising can trigger an adrenal crash. The more advanced the adrenal fatigue, the less vigorous the exercise should be.

One of the dangers of self-guided adrenal fatigue recovery programs is the tendency to over-exercise once more energy is regained. The body might not be ready to tolerate more strenuous exercise and can lead to a relapse. A person with advanced adrenal fatigue should not proceed with any exercise routine without professional supervision. Our tailor-made exercise routines will help incorporate the correct type and amount of exercise into your schedule to help with adrenal fatigue recovery.

Supplements for Adrenal Fatigue

Ashwagandha and Rhodiola — they are known to reduce stress and anxiety. Ashwagandha reduces cortisol levels, while Rhodiola reduces stress through regulating the neurotransmitter transport in the brain.

Vitamin C — This is another crucial supplement in adrenal function and maintenance of healthy levels of cortisol and DHEA. Deficiencies of this vitamin can have a profound effect on adrenal function.

Vitamin B2 and Vitamin B6 — B complex vitamins are important vitamins that act as coenzymes in various biochemical reactions in cells and regulate many processes in the body, such as cell metabolism. They assist in the production of various hormones in the adrenal gland, including cortisol, adrenaline, aldosterone, estrogen and testosterone, that help the body cope with stress. A deficiency in B vitamins leads to low energy levels and increased fatigue.

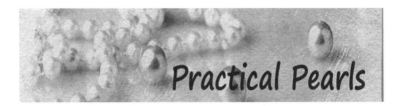

Practical Pearls

1.	Recognize the symptoms of stress and adrenal fatigue.
2.	Identify the causes for this stress; see the 7 C causes in my book, *The Heart of the Matter*.
3.	Remain steadfast in finding solutions to the causes of your stress.
4.	Modify your lifestyle to include adequate sleep, gentle exercise and good relaxation time.
5.	Learn some relaxation techniques, which can be used as needed.
6.	Eat a healthy diet.
7.	Take our supplement Reserene™ to help restore adrenal function.

2.4 Attitude

It is essential to develop a robust, positive and healthy attitude to life. You have to feel in control of your health and not a victim of the inevitable changes and deterioration that accompanies aging. There are a number of healthy lifestyle habits that can contribute to your health and anti-aging program. They will help to provide a feeling of wellness, as well as increase your strength and provide you with a sense of control. These include healthy eating, a good exercise program, sufficient sleep, reducing your stress levels and having purpose and fulfillment in your life.

The key anti-aging attitude is not to live out the program by feeling your age. Statements like "I am feeling my age"; "I am too old for that"; or "You go, I am way past my prime to do that activity" are all statements reinforcing the view that one has to slow down and get old. Instead, one needs to remove the perception of feeling old and do what's needed to be done.

Changing a lifestyle habit can be challenging, especially if you have been doing the same thing for many years. For example, we have seen the patient who has severe emphysema and although he has been strongly advised to stop smoking, he will not consider the idea — even with the known risk factors. We have also seen the patient who is high risk for a heart attack, but he refuses to change his diet or start an exercise program.

We now ask the question: What is the reason that people who know they are at risk for health complications do not change their lifestyle — even if they are told that doing so will save their life? To understand this dynamic, we need to understand the foundation for motivating a person. Motivation for experiencing pleasure or achieving success is obvious, because the result is experienced directly and provides a good feeling. But what motivates a person to exercise or stop eating pleasurable foods — if a person doesn't enjoy exercise and doesn't sense any tangible gain from eating the right foods?

The answer lies in the fact that one does not see a direct connection between the habit and the risk. Whilst someone is enjoying a plate of greasy French fries, it is difficult to understand intellectually that it is causing damage. If one could feel that each French fry actually causes direct damage to their health and that each step on the treadmill improves the walls of their blood vessels, it would be easier to change one's habits for the better.

The damage is not something that may happen in a few years, rather it occurs as you eat that specific serving of French fries. Chemical changes are occurring instantaneously as you eat, and these directly affect the blood vessels. And it is the same with exercise — the internal health benefit is immediate. One has to have a clear picture of the immediate effects of unhealthy habits, so that the greasy plate of French fries will become unappetizing, and the pleasure of feeling healthy will be more appealing. A person loses his desire to fly by jumping out of a 10-story window, because he sees the immediate effect of landing down below. In other words, if we clearly see the direct effects of taking on positive lifestyle choices and the negative consequences of unhealthy habits, we become motivated to adhere to these positive changes and lose the desire to return to our old, unhealthy ways.

So let's get going!

2.5 Sleep

Although sleep is a passive activity — and one that we do not give enough attention to — its benefits of allowing the brain and body to recover are enormous. Sleep helps facilitate the organization of the long-term memory and the integration of new information. Whilst REM sleep largely affects brain repair and restoration, non-REM sleep is mainly a time for body repair and renewal. There are automatic transformations that occur with sleep, including changes in brain waves, the restoration of hormone and chemical levels throughout the body, as well as the repair and renewal of tissues and nerve cells.

Insufficient sleep is implicated in the onset of degenerative diseases, which is associated with premature aging. Poor sleep also has a high correlation with the onset of Alzheimer's disease.

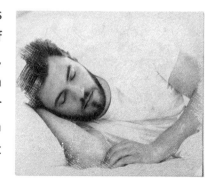

Our routine and habits that have a direct impact on our quality of sleep are often referred to as "sleep hygiene." Our daily schedule and actions, especially prior to going to bed, can impact how easy it is to fall asleep, stay asleep and feel refreshed when we wake up in the morning. Our health, brain function and mood are directly affected by the quality of sleep we get. Ensuring that we get the best quality and quantity of sleep per night is essential in helping our body recover and refresh itself.

Sleep Supplements

Pharma GABA — Gamma-aminobutyric acid (GABA) is a major neurotransmitter that is found in abundance and widely distributed throughout the central nervous system. Low levels of GABA function in the brain is associated with neurological disorders, most primarily anxiety, depression, and insomnia. A natural form of GABA has been manufactured using a fermentation process that utilizes Lactobacillus Hilgardii. It has been shown to induce relaxation by (a) increasing the alpha to beta brainwave ratio, (b) preserving salivary antibody production during stress, and (c) reducing markers of stress including cortisol levels.

Once ingested, it is absorbed easily and binds to GABA receptors in the peripheral nervous system. Usually within 5 to 30 minutes of ingestion, it activates the parasympathetic nervous system, which is responsible for producing what is referred to as the "relaxation response," a physiological response that is in direct contrast to the stress or fight-or-flight response. Studies with Pharma GABA have shown an impressive ability to improve sleep quality, enabling a person to feel refreshed and ready to tackle their day.

Valerian is a tall, flowering grassland plant that has demonstrated in multiple studies, the ability to reduce the amount of time it takes to fall asleep and help attain a deeper sleep. Clinical studies have shown that Valerian stimulates the brain's GABA receptor, a neurological gateway for sleep-inducing chemicals.

Passion flower is an herb that helps calm the nerves, reduces anxiety, helps with insomnia and soothes nervous tension. Studies have found that passion flower assists people in falling asleep more quickly and increases their quality of sleep.

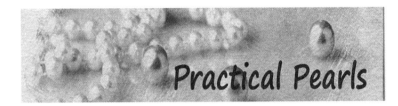

1. *Ensure that your bedroom is cool, quiet and dark. An important sleep-regulating hormone called melatonin, is enhanced when a person sleeps in a dark room with the shade and curtains drawn. Even a small amount of light reduces the melatonin output from our brains.*

2. *By going to sleep and waking up at more or less the same time each day, including weekends, it reinforces a schedule on the body's sleep-wake cycle and helps a person fall asleep more easily at night. It is also advantageous to create a wind-down routine before bedtime, such as taking a warm bath or shower, reading a book or listening to relaxing music.*

3. *It is preferable to avoid an adrenaline rush first thing in the morning. Therefore, turn off computers, smartphones and other devices that might trigger a shock to your system, and place alarms at least 10 feet away from the bed. It is also better to turn off night lights.*

4. *Avoid adrenal stimulants that impose excessive stress on the adrenal glands, such as sugary foods and caffeine – especially at night time – as they can interfere with sleep patterns. Nicotine and alcohol also have an adverse effect on sleep.*

5. *Our cortisol levels are lowered at night and it is therefore best to go to sleep before 10 p.m., so as not to push our bodies beyond their natural limits. In the years before the invention of electricity, people had no choice other than to go to bed when it was dark and awake at sunrise.*

6. *A light protein snack before bedtime can help promote sleep, for example, a handful of nuts or cottage cheese.*

7. *If you have trouble falling asleep, try and do some breathing exercises or relaxation techniques and go back to bed when you are tired. Don't agonize over falling asleep; it creates added stress.*

CHAPTER 3

PURPOSE AND SOCIAL CONTACT

PURPOSE

The opposite of having purpose may be defined as depression. If there is no feeling of a need to accomplish something, then life becomes pretty empty and meaningless. When we wake up in the morning, we may have something significant to accomplish that day, or we may have to think of how to keep busy to pass another day.

Purpose means that we have something unique to achieve or to give to others. This may include fulfilling a lifelong dream, such as learning a new skill, creating a piece of art or music, or even exploring something that we have always had a passion to do. In short, it means some form of self-development and growth.

Purpose can also be in the form of giving to others, whether through our knowledge and experience or through helping people less fortunate than us. It means making the lives of others better than they were before. Living a life without purpose would result in the constant search for instant thrills and gratification, such as gambling, or doing trivial tasks just to feel alive.

There is a greater risk of losing purpose when we reach retirement age or we no longer have a need to earn a living. We all dream about our retirement years, and yet it may be the most significant factor that contributes to aging. When we retire, we suddenly have excess free time on our hands and often replace an active lifestyle with hours of passive activity. Sitting in front of the TV, doing some shopping or watching sport are all passive pastimes and contribute to lackluster functioning and lead to dullness of the brain and other organs.

It has been proven that as we age, if we keep involved with meaningful activities and wake up in the morning with a purpose and an excitement, this will have a significant influence on our health and longevity. It will also have a positive effect on our brain functioning and memory. It is essential to seek real, important and meaningful activities to fill our lives. My book *Heart of the Matter* provides an in-depth explanation of this crucial area.

SOCIAL CONTACT

Social isolation has been proven to be a high-risk factor for chronic disease and early death. Frequent visits and contact with family and friends is crucial. If you feel you are being forgotten or neglected, then call up your family members or a friend and initiate contact. It is often our perception that people don't want to hear from us or are too busy for us, however in reality they are usually happy to reignite a relationship.

Casual relationships are also important. Speak to your neighbors, be friendly with the store owner down the block, join groups and sports clubs. People are usually happy when someone initiates a friendly conversation or at least a greeting.

The bottom line is don't build artificial walls around yourself and become isolated from society. The health benefits of being connected include a positive effect on brain health and certainly on mood and mental health. These in turn will have a positive influence on your general well-being. Remember, we only live once. Don't be embarrassed to get out, be with people and stay socially active.

CHAPTER 4

THE IMMUNE SYSTEM

The immune system consists of a sophisticated group of cells which react to foreign elements that enter the body. These elements can be in the form of infective agents, such as bacteria, viruses, parasites or fungi that lead to infection, as well as allergenic agents that result in allergies.

Upon invasion, cells known as T cells are activated by infective agents. Depending on the type of invader, one of two reactions will occur: either the T cell will activate a Th1 response, whereby macrophages (cells that can gobble up foreign invaders) will directly attack these foreign agents, or alternatively, a Th2 reaction will occur, whereby T cells set off a reaction leading to the production of antibodies that attack the invading agents. These antibodies are proteins that are specifically produced to attach to an invading agent and neutralize it.

If there is an overreaction of the Th1 system, it causes the immune system to attack parts of the body. This is usually organ specific, as in the case of Hashimoto's disease, which causes damage to the thyroid, or multiple sclerosis, which causes damage to the brain and spinal cord.

If there is an overreaction of the Th2 system, then more widespread autoimmune diseases occur, such as Lupus or scleroderma, which attack many systems. Allergies are also due to an overactive Th2 system.

The opposite of an overactive immune system is an underactive immune system. This weakness leaves the body unable to adequately fight infections, and recurrent or chronic viruses can result. For example, chronic sinusitis, frequent colds and viruses, or more severe infections that persist, such as pneumonia. A healthy immune system not only ensures a healthy response to eradicating and suppressing infections, it also prevents an overactive response of the immune system from spiraling out of control and causing damage to the body.

The body has a number of barriers that prevent foreign agents from entering its system and causing an immune or allergic response. The skin is the body's external barrier and the lining of the bowel, known as the epithelial lining, forms an internal barrier. It is essential to take good care of our skin and to keep the bowel epithelial layer healthy. Infections and allergies to foods and other substances can disrupt and damage the barrier, thereby allowing the entry of foreign agents. This in turn can cause an immune response that may lead to the development of more allergies or even autoimmune diseases.

The aim of our program is to reduce the exposure to allergens and infective agents and to create a healthy and balanced bowel function.

4.1 Inflammation

There is an additional way in which the body reacts to damage or infection. It is called the inflammatory response. Inflammation is a vital part of the body's immune response. It is the body's first line of defense to attempt to heal itself after an injury; defend itself against foreign invaders, such as viruses and bacteria; and repair damaged tissue.

When tissues are injured by bacteria, trauma, toxins, heat or any other causes, the damaged cells release inflammatory mediators, including histamine, bradykinin, and prostaglandins. They stimulate the narrow blood vessels in the tissue to expand, allowing more blood to reach the injured tissue. This causes the area to become red and hot.

Although inflammation initiates healing, ongoing chronic inflammation keeps the body on constant high alert and can in fact harm the body. It is characterized by the simultaneous repair and destruction of the tissue from the inflammatory process. Ongoing chronic inflammation will cause damage to other organs and tissues, including the brain, heart, blood vessels and other systems. It is important to find the root of the inflammation and treat it accordingly to prevent the onset of dangerous illness. Some people are hyper-inflamed, which is often associated with obesity. Taking control of your weight by adhering to a healthy diet will help control inflammation. Natural supplements, including Curcumin and Boswellia, are excellent anti-inflammatories and should be taken daily to curb inflammation.

Supplements for Inflammation

Curcumin — NF-κB controls many genes linked with inflammation and is notably active in many inflammatory diseases, such as inflammatory bowel disease, arthritis, sepsis, gastritis, asthma and atherosclerosis. Curcumin has long been known to have poor bioavailability, requiring high doses to achieve desired blood levels. Our supplement, curcumin meriva, contains a novel curcumin absorption system which has been developed to deliver up to seven times more pharmacologically bioactive curcumin to the blood compared with commercial curcumin products.

Boswellia — The resinous extract called olibanum is obtained from Boswellia tree species, which are grown in India, Ethiopia and the Arabian Peninsula. In the western world it is known as frankincense. This resin contains anti-inflammatory, anti-arthritic and analgesic properties and helps alleviate joint swelling in arthritis.

PQQ — Pyrroloquinoline quinone (PQQ) is a novel vitamin-like compound found in plant foods. PQQ is an important antioxidant that boosts the formation of new mitochondria, along with supporting heart health and cognitive function. Preclinical studies and initial clinical evaluations are showing a wide range of benefits to both brain and body function, which includes the regulation of cellular energy metabolism and the reduction of inflammation.

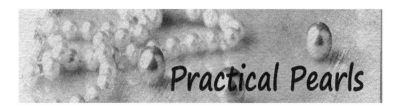

Practical Pearls

1. *Test for elevated markers of inflammation including Hs CRP, ferritin levels, CBC, vitamin D levels, omega 3 / omega 6 ratio (arachidonic acid).*

2. *Make sure you have a bi-yearly dental and hygiene check. Floss and brush your teeth and gums daily, and if there are signs of potential infection, have them treated.*

3. *Eat a low inflammatory diet – avoid fried foods, margarine and partially hydrogenated oils, sugar, refined flour and nightshade vegetables (potatoes, tomatoes, eggplant and peppers).*

4. *If there are any other potential infections, such as chronic diarrhea or chronic sinus pain, have them treated.*

5. *Do the appropriate testing if there are symptoms suggesting autoimmune diseases. This includes a blood panel for diseases such as Hashimoto's disease of the thyroid, inflammatory bowel disease like Crohn's disease or ulcerative colitis, joint disease like rheumatoid arthritis or psoriatic arthritis.*

6. *If any blood test results indicate an autoimmune disease, make sure you take a celiac test, which is often associated with autoimmune issues.*

7. *It is imperative to heal the gut and intestinal tract in order to slow down or prevent autoimmune disease, as gut problems can set off autoimmune complications.*

8. *Curcumin and Boswellia are very strong anti-inflammatory herbs that have many other health benefits as well. Try our Ignite product called Remobility.*™

4.2 Cancer Prevention

The development of cancer is also connected somewhat to the immune system. Abnormal precancerous cells evolve all the time and are eliminated by the immune system before they take root. There is a delicate balance between maintaining healthy cell growth and preventing senescence or aging, and over-stimulating cells which leads to cancer.

Various factors can lead to the over-stimulation of cancer cells, including genetic factors. Many people have genes that predispose them to cancer, which puts them in a higher risk category for developing the disease. However, these genes do not necessarily have to be expressed. A classic example is the BRCA 1 gene deletion, whereby people with this defect may have up to an 80% chance of developing breast cancer in their lifetime. But this does not have to be the case, because living a healthful life in all ways will prevent the expression of this gene.

Cancer does not only affect people who are predisposed to a defective gene, but typically occurs in people living an unhealthy lifestyle. The following are common issues that promote cancer:

- Smoking
- Toxins — particularly those found in processed meats, some processed foods, pesticides that are used to protect foods from bugs, some artificial hormones and contaminated nuts and grains
- Eating flame-broiled meat or meat charred on a barbecue

- Poor nutrition — this includes eating inflammatory provoking foods like sugars, refined carbohydrates, bad fats and partially hydrogenated oil, which is contained in fried foods, margarine and processed foods.
- Excess alcohol
- Stress — this has a high correlation with cancer incidence and is paramount to keep in control.
- Social isolation
- BPA, phthalates and other estrogens

CANCER PREVENTION STRATEGIES

It is important to take the necessary steps and do the correct screening to detect cancer in its early stages. There is routine screening for the general public and then there is more intensive screening for people who have a higher risk, such as those with a family history of cancer or a personal genetic risk for cancer. A physician can guide you with regard to the correct screening; make sure that you have a competent physician to manage your program. Although it is essential to do your screening program, do not become neurotic or hypochondriacal. If you live a healthy lifestyle and have a good robust attitude to life, you can do your tests as needed and then forget about being over-vigilant and anxious once you have passed the tests.

The following are strategies to prevent cancer:

1. *Exercise* — see the section on exercise. All forms of exercise are good.

2. *Maintain healthy nutrition* — this plays a vital role in preventing cancer.

❖ It is important to eat 10 servings of fruit and vegetables a day.
❖ Eat 100% whole grains/ increase fiber.
❖ Meat should be grass-fed, pasture-raised and organic. It must be slow-cooked and not burnt, cured or processed. Meat should be used sparingly and added to the main vegetable course.
❖ Incorporate fish into your diet, but no more than twice weekly and it should not be farmed fish. The following fish are recommended: salmon, mackerel, anchovy, sardine, herring.
❖ Poultry should be free range and organic.
❖ Avoid food additives and aspartame.
❖ Avoid all sugars and foods containing fructose (which is one of the most harmful foods).
❖ Eat healthy fats and avoid trans fat.
❖ Avoid fried food.

> ❖ Caloric restriction is becoming more popular in the fight against cancer growth.

3. *Maintain good levels of vitamin D* — aim for levels of about 50 ng/ml or more of vit D 25 OH.
4. *Incorporate omega-3 fish oil into your diet*— it has been proven to prevent breast cancer.
5. *The following nutraceuticals may help in preventing cancer:*

> ❖ Lycopene (the most effective prevention against prostate cancer)
> ❖ Korean ginseng
> ❖ Astaxanthin
> ❖ Fisetin
> ❖ Reishi mushroom
> ❖ Berberine
> ❖ Vitamin D
> ❖ Quercetin and tocotrienols (useful in eliminating senescent cells that contribute to cancer)
> ❖ Selenium 200 mcg (has a strong anti-cancer effect)

6. *Reduce stress*

CHAPTER 5

THE FUNCTIONAL SYSTEMS

In this section, you will find an overall description of the functioning of the major systems of the body. This will enable you to understand how they work and what is involved in maintaining them as part of a whole, healthy unit. Identifying early signs of weakness in a system is important in order to reverse the damage.

The weakness of one or more systems may be more relevant to one particular person than another, as every individual has their own pattern of strengths and weaknesses. This pattern is called an Age Print. Working with your Age Print will empower you to take early preventive measures to prevent the onset of chronic illnesses. There are tests for each system, and based on the results, you can determine weaknesses that require attention. The general testing for each system will be indicated in the following sections.

5.1 The Cardiovascular System

THE PUMP

The heart — which is located in the center of the chest cavity between the lungs — pumps blood to the lungs, where it releases carbon dioxide and becomes re-oxygenated. The oxygenated blood is then pumped back to the heart from where it is distributed around the body through the blood vessels. The muscle of the heart requires a good supply of blood in order to receive oxygen and produce energy. It also needs to contract and pump and relax in order to refill. As we age, our bodies change and slow down. The blood supply to the muscles is reduced due to the narrowing of the blood vessels and there may be a reduction in essential enzymes, minerals and nutrients required for the efficient pumping of the heart muscle.

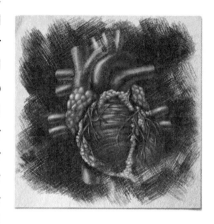

Our aim is to preserve a good blood supply to the heart muscle and provide it with essential nutrients, minerals and enzymes. The heart must also be kept in excellent working condition by adhering to a regular exercise routine and staying active.

A heartbeat is a single cycle in which your heart's chambers relax and contract to pump blood. The muscle is stimulated to pump by an electrical stimulus which is under the influence of the autonomic nervous system. Stress and anxiety influence this system negatively, and it is essential that the parasympathetic nervous system is dominant and stress is kept to a minimum. Dangerous arrhythmias and abnormal heart functioning can occur with ongoing stress and anxiety.

The best interventions for heart health are:

- Exercise
- Naturals supplements and minerals
- Avoiding stress and anxiety

There are a number of tests that can be performed to evaluate the effectiveness of your heart function. They include:

- Blood tests that assess the risk for damage to the arteries of the heart (the coronary arteries). These blood tests are the same tests to check for blood vessel health discussed in the next section.
- Echocardiogram — this test checks the heart muscle health and functioning and the health of the heart valves.
- If an irregular heartbeat or arrhythmia occurs, then an EKG or halter test needs to be done to identify what type of irregular beat exists, and how to treat it.
- Doing a heart rate variability (HRV) test is important, as this determines whether the sympathetic nervous system is affecting the heart. If the heart rhythm is very regular — in other words, there is very little variability in the rhythm — it means that there is too much influence from the sympathetic nervous system on the heart. This is the stress system and has a major negative effect on the functioning of the heart.

The following supplements are important for heart health:

Coenzyme Q10 (COQ10): This is a nutrient produced in the body that helps mitochondria produce energy. A decline in COQ10 levels causes tissues to burn fuel inefficiently, resulting in oxidative damage and eventually loss of function. A deficiency and the resulting bioenergetic collapse are the underlying causes of heart failure, one of the leading causes of death and disability in the world today. COQ10 is recommended for people suffering from heart disease or fibromyalgia, as these diseases are associated with low COQ10 levels.

Magnesium is among the top nutrients for heart health. It is used in a number of enzymatic reactions and is necessary for normal muscle function, helping to maintain smooth muscle function in the blood vessels. A shortage can cause or worsen congestive heart failure, atherosclerosis, chest pain, high blood pressure, cardiac arrhythmias, heart muscle disease (cardiomyopathy), heart attack and even sudden cardiac death.

Hawthorn, which has been shown to exhibit antioxidant capabilities, contains valuable flavonoids in the leaves, berries, and blossoms. One of these flavonoids, proanthocyanidin, is especially relevant for cardiovascular health. It has the ability to increase coronary arterial blood flow, perhaps due to dilation of the coronary arteries. Hawthorn also appears to slightly increase the strength of the cardiac muscle contractions and decrease blood pressure, resulting in increased exercise tolerance and protection against congestive heart failure.

Arjuna is one of the most popular and beneficial medicinal plants in the treatment of cardiovascular diseases. It has shown promising success in decreasing the persistence of angina attacks, as well as stimulating healthy heart function and assisting with the regeneration of the heart muscles.

5.2 The Supply Lines — The Circulatory System

Blood is pumped around the body to all tissues and organs

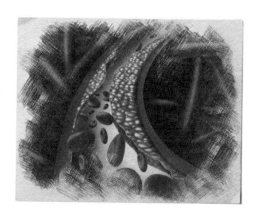

via a complex network of blood vessels, including arteries, veins and capillaries. It is propelled through the arteries by the pressure generated from the heartbeat. Generally, arteries transport oxygenated blood from the lungs to the body and its organs, and veins transport deoxygenated blood from around the body back to the heart. It is important to keep all the bloods vessels clean and functioning well to ensure the normal passageway and circulation of blood.

There are two areas of the bloods vessels that need to be maintained in excellent condition. The endothelium, or the inner layer of the blood vessels, and the muscle layer of the vessels.

If the endothelium is damaged, it allows abnormal substances and cells to enter the inner lining of the vessels. Excess LDL (low-density-lipoprotein) cholesterol that enters the subendothelial layer have a high chance of becoming oxidized, causing an immune response to occur. The immune cells recognize these oxidized LDL particles as being foreign invaders, and they swallow them up and create foam cells that make up the plaque that narrows the arteries. Over time, the plaque can cause clotting in the narrow section of the artery and result in a heart attack or stroke.

There are many causes of endothelial damage, including excess inflammation, toxins, insufficient essential minerals and vitamins, excess glucose, abnormal lipids such as small dense LDL cholesterol and inadequate quantities of the large fluffy HDL cholesterol particles. The large fluffy HDL cholesterol particles help prevent buildup of plaque in the arteries by carrying the dangerous LDL cholesterol back to the liver.

When calculating your cholesterol levels, it is important to remember that it is not enough to know your total cholesterol number; you also need to know the number of LDL particles and the size of these particles. If there is a high particle number with small dense LDL particles, then there is a greater risk for developing atherosclerosis. The size and number of your LDL and HDL cholesterol can be measured using an advanced lipid test, and the results can be interpreted by your physician.

Smoking is also a big contributing factor to cardiovascular disease and causes constriction and damage to the blood vessels and small arterioles that supply the kidney, brain and other organs. This in turn can damage these organs.

Metabolic syndrome is another factor that causes vessel damage. However, it is often a forgotten risk factor and many people and even physicians are hooked on beating down cholesterol levels, whilst ignoring this very significant component.

The metabolic syndrome is caused by a number of risk factors that together result in a phenomenon called insulin resistance. When we eat food, our blood sugar levels rise. Cells in the pancreas are signaled to release insulin into the bloodstream. Insulin then attaches to and signals cells to absorb sugar from the bloodstream, which in turn lowers the blood sugar levels.

Insulin resistance occurs when the pancreas secretes increasing amounts of insulin into the bloodstream but the cells in the tissues have become resistant and do not react. Higher levels of insulin together with high levels of glucose remain in the blood, which is in itself toxic to the body. The pancreas is overworked and starts to fail, and then Type 2 diabetes sets in. All of this causes damage to the blood vessels.

The causes of the metabolic syndrome are:

- High blood pressure
- Elevated blood glucose
- Overweight - too much fat tissue especially abdominal fat (a large belly)
- High triglycerides- these are fats mainly produced from excess sugars and carbohydrates in the diet
- Low HDL cholesterol - this is the good cholesterol

If you have 3 out of 5 of these risk factors, then you have the metabolic syndrome. The treatment is as follows:

- Decrease sugars and carbs in your diet
- Lose weight
- Exercise
- Keep good blood pressure control

The muscular layer of the arteries is considered healthy when it is elastic and not stiff. Stiffness of the arteries will cause an increase in blood pressure and result in further damage to the arteries and essential organs. The heart will have to pump against stiff, non-compliant arteries and will need to work much harder.

Therefore, high blood pressure is really a sign of damage to the arterial blood vessels. The blood pressure is a measure of the pressure that the heart exerts when it pumps, i.e., the systolic blood pressure, and the pressure in the arteries when the heart relaxes, i.e., the diastolic blood pressure. It is important to maintain good blood pressure levels at every age, as even a slight increase has been shown to have bad effects on the heart, the kidneys and other organs. A normal blood pressure is 120/80 or less. It is essential to visit your physician if your blood pressure constantly fluctuates.

Strategies to decrease high blood pressure include:

- Exercising on most days
- Reducing stress
- Ensuring that you have good quality sleep
- Maintaining a healthy diet

The following supplements are helpful to reduce blood pressure:

Hawthorn berry has been shown to promote blood flow in smaller vessels, as well as reduce blood pressure, much like ACE inhibitors. It also helps to ease angina and relieve congestive heart failure.

Celery seeds contain potassium, which helps to lower blood pressure by flushing sodium from the body via the kidneys. They have a high natural nitrite content, which have a blood pressure lowering effect by dilating blood vessels.

Olive leaf extract contains oleuropein, which is a compound that is found in high concentration levels in the olive leaf. It has been shown to favorably modulate high blood pressure's core mechanism, namely, arterial resistance or stiffness. Studies have shown that olive leaf extract supplements can bring about a significant reduction in blood pressure.

Seaweed — According to research published in the American Chemical Society's Journal of Agricultural and Food Chemistry, wakame (and other edible seaweeds) is a rich source of proteins that are known as bioactive peptides. They have a similar effect to ACE inhibitor drugs, which are widely prescribed to help lower blood pressure and prevent heart attacks and strokes.

Green coffee is derived from extracts of green, unroasted coffee that are high in chlorogenic acids. Studies have shown that the supplementation of green coffee bean extract improves both systolic and diastolic blood pressure levels.

Tests for arterial health include the following:

- Check for inflammation with HS CRP, ferritin level.

- Check lipids in the blood with an advanced lipid profile, which includes the LDL size and particle number, the HDL size and particle number, LPa.

- Check for signs of the metabolic syndrome which causes insulin resistance and leads to diabetes and blood vessel damage. Check triglycerides, blood pressure, waist circumference, fasting glucose and fasting insulin levels.

- Check the homocysteine level, which is a breakdown product of protein. If it is high, it indicates the body's inability to eliminate toxins, and this can cause vessel damage.

- Check if there is microalbumin in the urine, as this is associated with early kidney damage and vascular disease.

- Do an endopath test, which assesses endothelial health and elasticity of the muscles of the vessels.

- Do a carotid doppler, which is a specialized ultrasound of the main artery going to the neck, where one can see the intimal medial thickness and if there is plaque buildup. This correlates with the status of the other blood vessels.

These tests will have to be ordered and interpreted by a health provider who is experienced in functional medicine or anti-aging medicine, and who can provide solutions for any abnormalities.

Arterial health is therefore critical in order to maintain healthy essential organs. It is achieved through the same strategies that help to reduce blood pressure, namely:

- ❖ Sufficient exercise
- ❖ Healthy diet
- ❖ Supplements that are appropriate for blood vessel health
- ❖ Stress prevention

Supplements include the following ingredients:

Pomegranate — Packed with unique antioxidants and anti-inflammatory effects, pomegranate has shown promising results in both laboratory and clinical studies in averting various pathological changes associated with cardiovascular disease. Its antioxidant compounds have also been shown to reduce blood pressure naturally. Scientists believe that pomegranate works via several mechanisms to fight heart disease by

- reducing oxidative stress,

- supporting the synthesis and activity of nitric oxide,

- inhibiting the oxidation of potentially harmful LDL (low-density lipoproteins, or bad cholesterol).

Pine bark Extract — Pine Bark Extract (also known as Pycnogenol) is a natural plant extract originating in the bark of the Maritime Pine. It is found to contain a unique combination of procyanidins, bioflavonoids and organic acids, which are excellent free-radical scavengers. It is also known as a powerful antioxidant that is high in oligomeric proanthocyanidin compounds (OPCs), which are antibacterial, anti-aging and anticarcinogenic. Clinical studies have shown Pycnogenol to help maintain vascular function and support a healthy, balanced inflammatory response.

Grape seed extract - The latest findings demonstrate that full-spectrum grape seed extract can help support cardiovascular health by maintaining youthful endothelial function, regulating the clumping together of platelets in the blood and reducing inflammation. Blood vessel lining cells (endothelial cells) are charged with maintaining muscle tone and smoothness of arterial walls, thereby controlling blood pressure and the tendency for plaques to form and platelets to congregate. It is becoming increasingly clear that reducing lipid peroxidation-induced damage to delicate endothelial cells is an important way to maintain vascular health. There are several mechanisms at work here, including the production of the important signaling molecules nitric oxide and endothelin-1, both of which are beneficially affected by grape seed polyphenols.

Olive leaf extract — Olive leaf extract contains oleuropein, a natural compound, which is an antioxidant and anti-inflammatory that has disease fighting characteristics. It supports healthy blood pressure, and therefore, healthy blood flow and vessels.

5.3 The G.I. System

BREAKDOWN AND ABSORPTION OF FOOD

The gastrointestinal system is the largest organ in the body and pertains to the mouth, esophagus, stomach and intestines. This system takes in food, digests it to extract and absorb nutrients and expels the remaining waste as feces. Infective agents like bacteria and viruses are also eliminated through the GI tract. There are many aspects of the GI tract that need to be cared for in order to ensure a smooth functioning system.

The GI tract consists of trillions of bacteria known as the microbiota, which play a crucial role in gut health as well as the immune system. Therefore, keeping a healthy balance of these bacteria is very important. An individual's makeup of gut microbiota is established at birth, although it changes throughout life according to age, location, food and supplement intake and other environmental influences.

Taking the correct probiotics and prebiotics can assist the gut microbiota and improve a person's gut health.

The stomach requires adequate gastric acid for digestion. At the same time, you do not want this acid to reflux up the esophagus (known as gastroesophageal reflux) which can damage it. When a person experiences heartburn or acid reflux, the first course of action is to reach for medication. This form of relief should only be used to heal the esophagus, after which time a more natural path should be taken to maintain the stomach acid level and to control reflux.

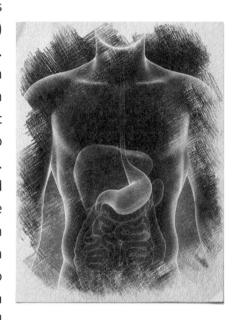

Additionally, sufficient digestive enzymes are needed to digest different food types, including fats, proteins and carbohydrates. Insufficient enzymes cause intestinal symptoms like flatulence, diarrhea and abdominal pains. This usually begins an hour or more after eating. Digestive enzymes can be replaced by means of supplements until they are produced by the intestines again.

Food allergies can also cause reactions in the intestines and disrupt the normal functioning of the bowel. Two tests can be performed to check for allergies to foods: (a) IgE testing, which detects recent exposure to an allergen; and (b) IgG testing, which has a longer memory and can detect exposure to an allergen from some time ago. Food allergies can develop any time in your life and is not age specific. If after eating a certain item you notice a change in how you feel, you break out in hives or your throat begins to itch, make an appointment with an allergist to be tested.

Another intestinal issue can occur when bacterial overgrowth develops in the small intestine (SIBO). SIBO results when bacteria from the large intestine spreads into the small intestine. This is a very unfavorable situation, as the large and the small intestines have different types and amount of bacteria growth. SIBO is treated with a combination of antibiotics and probiotics.

The attainment of GI health therefore involves the following:

- Maintaining adequate gastric acid in the stomach
- Cultivating sufficient intestinal enzymes in the small intestine
- Removing food allergens from your diet
- Removing chronic infections from the bowel
- Cultivating a good balance of healthy bacteria in the GI tract
- Having sufficient bowel movements to eliminate waste products by eating enough fiber and drinking enough fluids

A strong, robust gastrointestinal system requires an optimal diet for healthy functioning. You may need to supplement with hydrochloric acid and digestive enzymes and take the necessary steps to correct the distribution of bacteria in the gut.

A formula to help strengthen the gastrointestinal system should include the following ingredients:

Zinc carnosine — Zinc carnosine is a combination of the mineral zinc and the amino peptide L-carnosine that is renowned for soothing and supporting stomach health. The mucosal lining in the stomach is protected from its own gastric acid by a thin layer of gel-like mucus. Zinc carnosine is not easily broken down by these harsh gastric juices and is therefore able to strengthen the mucosal barrier by adhering to the stomach wall. The benefits include alleviating indigestion without suppressing the stomach acid that could affect digestion, as well as relieving symptoms of nausea, heartburn, bloating and belching.

Slippery elm bark (Ulmus rubra) and marshmallow root (Althea officinalis) contain mucilaginous components that are soothing to the digestive tract.

Mastic gum powder — Mastic contains antioxidants and also has antibacterial and antifungal properties. It has shown promising results in treating stomach and intestinal ulcers when taken over a two-week period. It may also ease gastritis and upset stomach, as well as decrease inflammation in the gastrointestinal tract.

Enzyme blend — This provides the body with enzymes designed to optimally aid the digestion of fats, proteins and carbohydrates presented in cooked and raw food. As we get older, the production of these vital enzymes diminishes, and it is important to supplement in order to maintain healthy digestion.

Enhanced super digestive enzymes — This includes specific enzymes needed to support the natural reactions that break down food and optimize digestion and nutrient absorption. Below is the broad array of enzymes contained in this formula:

- Protease enzymes help break down proteins.
- Amylase enzymes help break down starch and short sugar chains, called oligosaccharides.
- Lipase helps break down fats.
- Cellulase helps break down the indigestible polysaccharide in dietary cellulose.

5.4 The Liver

The liver is an organ in the body that supports almost every other organ in the body through its diverse roles.

1. Firstly, it is the center for detoxification and breakdown of waste products, whereby toxic ammonia, which is a byproduct of metabolism in the body, is converted to urea and is excreted via the kidneys in our urine.
2. The liver is also a storage organ where excess glucose is converted to fats and stored, and then later released into the blood as needed.

3. It breaks down excess toxins, insulin and hormones that are not needed through a number of metabolic processes.
4. Old red blood cells are broken down in the liver and removed through the intestines.
5. The liver produces bile, an alkaline compound that helps with the breakdown of fats, which assists with digestion.
6. The liver also produces cholesterol, proteins and clotting factors.

The liver cells are the factories where all this activity takes place, and it is therefore vital not to overburden them with toxins. Drugs such as paracetamol, non-steroidal anti-inflammatory drugs, certain cancer medication and many more drugs may damage these liver cells. Excessive alcohol 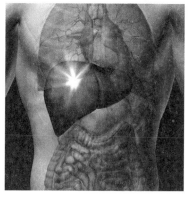 consumption also results in alcoholic liver disease, including alcoholic hepatitis, fatty liver and cirrhosis. Factors contributing to the development of alcoholic liver diseases are not only the quantity and frequency of alcohol consumption, but also include gender and genetics.

A poor diet comprised of sugars and carbohydrates causes excess fat buildup in the cells, which eventually damages them. Fructose, which is another form of sugar, is found in thousands of food products and sugary drinks. When it enters the liver, it kicks off a series of complex chemical transformations. One remarkable change is that the liver uses fructose, a carbohydrate, to create fat — a process called lipogenesis. Too much fructose causes tiny fat droplets to accumulate in liver cells, which is similar to what happens in the liver of people who drink too much alcohol. This is known as fatty liver disease, which can be reversed if treated sufficiently early.

Many chemicals may also affect the liver, including phthalates and BPA from plastics, as well as chemicals from insect and worm repellents on fruit and vegetables.

Due to its central role in supporting the overall functioning of most organs in the body, it is essential to maintain healthy liver function by taking the following supplements:

Milk thistle works in a number of ways to protect your liver on a daily basis. It contains silymarin, an antioxidant that protects the liver from toxins and drugs that cause liver damage. Silymarin reduces liver inflammation by inhibiting enzymes, such as 5-LOX, COX, and NFkB, that produce inflammatory cytokines and other harmful signaling molecules that can cause liver damage. It has also been shown to prevent liver fibrosis — the first step in the last stage of advanced liver disease — by protecting normal liver structural cells and blocking them from turning into fibrous, muscle-like cells.

N-A-C is a form of the essential amino acid cysteine, which is used by the body to make glutathione (GSH), one of the body's most important antioxidants. In fact, all the benefits of N-A-C arise from its ability to boost a person's GSH levels in the blood. N-A-C protects the body from many different toxins because of its content of sulfhydryl groups that can bind and inactivate herbicides, mercury, cadmium, lead, toxic heavy metals, drugs such as acetaminophen, environmental pollutants, microbes like E. Coli, carbon tetrachloride and aflatoxin.

There is a common condition known as non-alcoholic fatty liver disease (NAFLD). This condition enables the liver to store excessive amounts of fat, mostly due to insulin resistance, metabolic syndrome or diabetes. Liver function tests are usually elevated, indicating damage to liver cells, and the liver appears grossly fatty on an ultrasound. Studies show a significant improvement in liver function tests in those suffering from NAFLD with supplementation of N-A-C. Not only does it protect liver cells, but it also helps heal a damaged liver.

Schisandra chinensis is known as a liver "tonic" in traditional Chinese medicine, and appears to offer both a preventative and rehabilitative liver protection effect. It helps boost antioxidant activity, increase enzyme production, improve circulation and digestion and has the ability to assist with removing waste from the body.

Activated broccoli sprout extract is a well-known cruciferous vegetable superfood, with the sprouts being 20–150 times more nutrient-dense than the full grown plant. Research has shown that sulforaphane from broccoli has many profound health benefits, above and beyond helping the body with detoxification. Activated broccoli sprout extract helps improve and maintain liver function through reduction of oxidative stress.

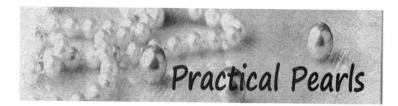

1. *Check over-the-counter and prescription medication information leaflets for potential liver damage, and avoid using if possible – examples are acetaminophen, statin drugs for high cholesterol and antifungal medication.*

2. *Drink alcohol in moderation, maximum 2 glasses of wine for men and 1 glass for women per day. If liver enzymes are elevated, then avoid alcohol altogether.*

3. *Avoid sugars and high carbohydrate foods and foods containing fructose.*

4. *Get plenty of exercise and keep your weight under control.*

5. *Avoid toxins in pesticides, cleansers, paints and solvents.*

6. *Avoid food in plastic containers, especially if they are heated in the microwave.*

7. *Use liver support products, including Milk Thistle and N-acetyl Cysteine (NAC).*

5.5 The Brain and Nervous System

If the brain is like a computer that controls all the functions of your body, then the nervous system is a network that sends messages back and forth from the brain to all parts of the body. The nervous system is made up of trillions of nerve cells originating in the brain and extending down the spinal cord and branching out with thread-like nerves to all organs and body parts. The nerve cells communicate with each other by transmitting chemicals called neurotransmitters, which attach to neuroreceptors on the adjacent nerve cell. These chemicals initiate various actions in the next cell, thereby procuring a particular reaction. For example, when you touch a hot kettle, the nerves in your skin shoot a message of pain to your brain. The brain then sends a message to your muscles to pull your hand away.

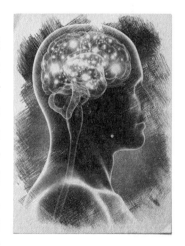

The brain requires sufficient neurotransmitters to function effectively. There are four important neurotransmitters required, as follows: dopamine, which is needed for attention, assertiveness and concentration; acetylcholine, which is needed for memory; GABA, which is needed for relaxing; and serotonin, which is needed to prevent depression. A deficiency in any of the above four neurotransmitters will result in symptoms related to that deficiency. Excess of the neurotransmitters can also produce symptoms including certain psychiatric problems.

Brain cells can be damaged irreversibly, and when a protein called amyloid builds up in the brain, it leads to Alzheimer's disease. Recently, a new concept was presented by the world-renowned expert on Alzheimer's treatment, Dr. Dale Bredesen, who discovered that the build-up of amyloid is a protective mechanism for the brain. This is in response to the three major insults to the brain: inflammation; the build-up of toxins; and the deficiency of certain vital vitamins, minerals and hormones. He has shown — in the laboratory and subsequently in patients — that by reversing these three damaging processes, one can reverse early Alzheimer's disease. It is possible nowadays to do extensive testing to identify which areas are weak and in need of correction.

The spinal cord consists of a long bundle of nerve tissue that extends from the lower part of the brain down through the spine. Various nerves branch out from the spine to the entire body along which messages are sent. These nerves make up the peripheral nervous system.

A part of the peripheral nervous system, called the **autonomic nervous system,** is responsible for controlling many of the body processes we almost never need to think about, like breathing, digestion, sweating and shivering. The autonomic nervous system has two parts: the sympathetic, or fight-or-flight response, and the parasympathetic, or rest-

and-digest nervous systems. They have been discussed above.

Therefore, to maintain an optimal nervous system we need to keep the brain functioning well by keeping it stimulated and making sure that our neurotransmitters are in top form. In addition, we have to be sure that the damaging processes leading to Alzheimer's disease are reversed. It has been proven lately that the preservation of brain cells and brain function can be greatly enhanced by the lifestyle factors contained in the Practical Pearls that follow. The following natural supplements have also been shown to help preserve brain cells and enhance brain function.

Brain Supplements

Lion's Mane — This is a beautiful, edible mushroom that grows like a white waterfall of cascading icicles on broad-leaf trees and logs. The subject of recent studies, Lion's Mane is renowned for providing support to the brain and nervous system. It is an NGF activator, which is essential for nerve growth, maintenance and survival.

Bacopa — The supplement Bacopa monnieri has been shown to improve memory formation and cognition by reducing anxiety. It interacts with the dopamine and serotonergic systems, however, its main mechanism concerns promoting neuron communication. This is achieved by increasing the growth of nerve endings called dendrites, which enhances the rate at which the nervous system communicates.

Fisetin — This supplement has positive effects on a number of common pathways associated with age-associated neurological diseases. This combination of actions suggests that fisetin has the potential to maintain brain function even in the presence of the diverse factors that contribute to the development of age-associated neurological diseases. Importantly, multiple studies in animal models suggest that fisetin can reduce the impact of age-related neurological diseases, especially those associated with cognitive deficits such as Alzheimer's disease.

Magnesium threonate — It has now been discovered that magnesium is a critical player in the activation of nerve channels that are involved in synaptic plasticity. This means that magnesium is critical for the physiological events that are fundamental to the processes of learning and memory. As it turns out, one form of magnesium, magnesium threonate, has the unique ability to permeate the blood brain barrier and help increase the protein that stimulates the growth of new brain cells.

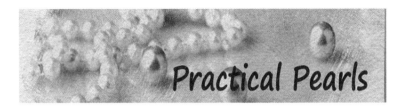

Practical Pearls

1. *Eating the correct nutrients and eliminating toxic foods from your diet can have an up to 30% reduction in the risk for dementia. One of the best-known diets for brain health and to prevent the onset of dementia and Alzheimer's disease is the MIND diet, which is a simple eating program that includes brain-healthy foods and precludes unhealthy choices.*

2. *Keep the brain "well oiled" with brain nutrients, including healthy fats and oils, omega-3 fatty acids and coconut oil, etc.*

3. *Regular exercise has also been proven to have a powerful preventive effect on brain dysfunction.*

4. *The brain is like any organ in the body – it needs to be well maintained by means of stimulation. It is important to keep the brain intellectually involved with brain activities, such as learning a new language or career.*

5. *Social isolation contributes to brain dysfunction and has been associated with an increased incidence of dementia. Keep yourself socially active and involved in community activities.*

6. *Retirement, vegetating in front of a TV, and allowing your brain to become a passive*

> *instrument are all strong risk factors for brain deterioration.*

7. *It is very important to have meaning and direction in your life and to wake up each day with a purpose of accomplishing something meaningful; see my book, Heart of the Matter.*

8. *Prevent stress – it is a big cause of Alzheimer's.*

9. *Make sure you get enough sleep.*

5.6 The Kidney or Renal System

The kidneys act as a filter to remove waste products and excess fluid from the body through the urine. The production of urine involves highly complex steps of excretion and reabsorption, which are necessary to maintain a stable balance of body minerals and salts.

The regulation of the body's salt, potassium and acid content is performed by the kidneys. The kidneys also produce hormones that affect the function of other organs, for example a hormone that stimulates red blood cell production and hormones that regulate blood pressure and control calcium metabolism.

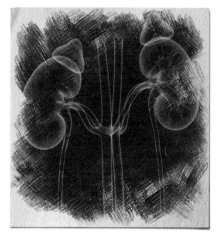

The kidneys are very sensitive organs and require a good blood flow at all times. The blood vessels supplying the kidneys need to be kept in healthy shape. There are many factors that may cause kidney damage, including excess use of over-the-counter medications, the most common being non-steroidal anti inflammatories, NSAIDS or drugs such as heroin and crack. Diabetes and high blood pressure are the most common causes of kidney disease, as well as excess lipids, which can also be detrimental.

Albumin is a type of protein found in large amounts in the blood. Because it is such a small molecule, it is one of the first proteins able to pass through the kidneys into the urine when there are kidney problems. When this is detected, immediate action must be taken to prevent the progression of further kidney problems. Drugs called ace inhibitors or angiotensin 2 receptor blockers are very helpful to prevent or lessen proteinuria (protein in the urine). Omega-3 oils and alpha lipoic acid are excellent supplements for the kidneys. Another toxic material that jeopardizes the kidneys is Cadmium, a soft metal that is highly toxic and can cause severe damage. If this is detected in the body, then a detox program must be used to treat this.

The prostate gland is a gland that is found in males and is situated after the bladder. The urethra is a tube that passes through the prostate and carries urine from the bladder to the outside. With age, the prostate can increase in size and constrict the urethra, resulting in a weak urinary stream. It also increases the urge to pass urine frequently. This condition is called benign prostatic hyperplasia BPH, and although it is not dangerous, it can cause a lot of discomfort and suffering. Another condition that affects the prostate is prostate cancer. Adequate screening should be done to prevent this aggressive type of cancer from occurring.

There are certain natural supplements which help to prevent prostatic enlargement and urinary symptoms. These include:

Lycopene is a naturally occurring chemical that gives fruits and vegetables a red color. This phytonutrient and carotenoid inhibits androgen receptor expression in prostate cancer cells and helps reduce prostate cancer cell proliferation. In a long-term study of about 14,000 participants, investigators found that men who ate five or more servings of tomatoes or tomato products each week, had a significantly lower risk of developing prostate cancer than men who consumed less than one serving per week.

Saw palmetto, which is found in south-east America, is a palm-like plant that has serrated, saw-like leaves and yellow berries that turn black when dried. Originally used by Native Americans, saw palmetto is a traditional herbal remedy used to relieve the symptoms of urinary tract conditions in men with an enlarged prostate (BPH).

Rye pollen extract has been shown to be effective at shrinking prostates enlarged by BPH and chronic prostatitis, and helps to reduce dangerous lower urinary tract symptoms that occur as a result. A study conducted in men with BPH concluded that those treated with the pollen extract were 2.4 times more likely to experience an improvement compared with those receiving a placebo. It also helped to reduce their need to urinate at night.

Pygeum Africanum Bark contains beneficial phytosterols that exhibit anti-inflammatory properties by inhibiting the production of prostaglandins in the prostate. It also contains ferulic esters, which reduce levels of prolactin (a hormone that promotes testosterone uptake in the prostate gland)

and pentacyclic triterpenes, which inhibit an enzyme involved in inflammation. Scientists believe that these phytochemicals work together to help counteract the structural and biochemical changes associated with benign prostatic hyperplasia.

Stinging nettle is a perennial flowering plant that is effective at relieving symptoms such as reduced urinary flow, incomplete emptying of the bladder, post urination dripping and the constant urge to urinate. These symptoms are caused by the enlarged prostate gland pressing on the urethra (the tube that empties urine from the bladder).

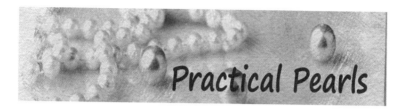

Practical Pearls

1. *Drink plenty of fluids throughout the day both in the summer and the winter months. Add a slice of lemon to water to add a refreshing flavor.*

2. *Maintain excellent blood glucose and cholesterol levels.*

3. *Maintain a normal blood pressure.*

4. *Avoid taking any drugs that may damage the kidneys – the most common being NSAIDS — non steroidal anti-inflammatory medication.*

5. *Live in a stress-free mode so that normal cortisol levels are maintained.*

6. *Take supplements that support kidney health.*

5.7 The Musculoskeletal System

The musculoskeletal system comprises the bones, muscles, tendons and ligaments. They are the support system for the whole body and are designed for movement and general physical functioning.

The bones are hard and made of calcium and other minerals. There are cells in the bones called osteoblasts that build new bone, as well as cells called osteoclasts that break down bone. As we age, our bones start to lose minerals and break down, which can lead to osteoporosis. Osteoporosis occurs either when we lose too much bone, don't make enough bone or a combination of both. This in turn predisposes people to fractures, other physical disabilities and even death. It is therefore crucial to ensure that we maintain healthy, strong bones.

The following are risk factors for osteoporosis that you can control:

- **Diet** — A diet that is low in vitamin D and calcium can contribute to weak bones. Vegetables such as broccoli and cauliflower, as well as dairy products, are a good source of calcium. The sun is a natural source of vitamin D, however, in order to get adequate amounts of vitamins necessary to preserve strong bones, you may need to take supplements.
- **Exercise** — High impact exercises, as well as strength training are important for maintaining muscle and bone strength into old age. Running, hiking, dancing and

weight-lifting are all good examples of exercises that build strong bones.

- **Smoking and alcohol consumption** — Research suggests that smoking and alcohol can negatively impact bone growth.
- **Medications** — Long term use of corticosteroids (such as prednisone and cortisone) have been associated with osteoporosis. Medication that suppresses stomach acid can also predispose you to osteoporosis, like protein pump inhibitors such as omeprazole.

The following are risk factors for osteoporosis that are beyond your control:

- Family history
- Female gender
- Ethnicity (Caucasians and Asians are at a higher risk)
- Body frame (smaller people have less bone)
- Age (the risk increases as you get older)

It is imperative to take sufficient minerals and vitamins to help build strong bones. There are a number of vitamins necessary for the absorption of calcium and minerals, including Vitamin D which needs to remain high at between 40-50 IU. Vitamin K2 is also important to direct calcium into the bones. A deficiency can result in calcium settling in the walls of blood vessels and in the heart valves, which can lead to severe heart valve or heart vessel disease. Vitamin K1 is converted to vitamin K2 in the gut, however it is preferable to take supplements of vitamin K2 at a dosage of 90–180 mcg a day.

Good hormone balance also contributes to bone health. These include estrogen, progesterone and some testosterone in females, and testosterone in males. As we age, and especially during menopause, these hormones dwindle and bone loss accelerates, which is why managing your hormone levels is crucial during this period in your life.

Other minerals that are good for bone strength are magnesium, manganese, boron, zinc. ReBone™, our vitamin supplement which was developed with the intention of preventing the onset and progression of osteoporosis, has been specially formulated with vitamins and minerals that are crucial for bone-building and bone-care. It is critical to build strong, dense bones whilst you are young and to keep them strong and healthy as you age.

Osteoblasts, which are responsible for the production of bone, need to be stimulated. Research has shown that when collagen is present in the bone matrix, it helps boost the activity of the osteoblasts, which need to be stimulated instead of osteoclasts. This is done primarily with exercise and most importantly, strength exercises. Regular strength training helps to deposit minerals in the bone muscles, thereby stimulating the osteoblasts.

Muscles are a greatly neglected tissue. The natural process as we age is that the muscles weaken and atrophy. However, even at a young age, if we do not use our muscles, they degenerate and are replaced by fat tissue. Fat tissue is unhealthy and causes increased inflammation in the body and can lead to insulin resistance and diabetes. Strong muscles on the other hand, are metabolically active and burn calories even when we sleep. It is essential to maintain muscle strength and functionality by means of exercise, especially strength training, which can be started at any age.

A healthy, balanced diet consisting of fresh fruits and vegetables, especially yellow and leafy green vegetables that are high in calcium, helps build strong bones. Foods that are rich in bone-protective antioxidants, such as broccoli, parsley and cabbage, help build strong bones in young adults and protect bone mass in old age.

Supplements for Preventing Sarcopenia

Vitamin D — While scientists have long known that vitamin D plays an important role in bone health, recent studies suggest that it is also essential for maintaining muscle mass in aging people. It has also recently been linked to muscle and bone tissue support and that low levels in older adults may be associated with poor bone and muscle function. Vitamin D helps preserve the Type II muscle fibers that are prone to atrophy in the elderly. Therefore, making sure you have sufficient vitamin D levels may help reduce the incidence of both osteoporosis and sarcopenia in aging people.

Leucine — Healthy muscles require amino acids, and leucine is one of the most important. It has the potential to maintain skeletal muscle protein synthesis and curb losses in muscular strength during the aging process.

Omega-3 powder — Fish oil-derived n-3 PUFA therapy, slows the normal decline in muscle mass and function in older adults and helps prevent sarcopenia. Recent human studies demonstrate that omega-3 fatty acids of marine origin can influence the metabolic and functional response of the skeletal muscle to exercise and nutrition. Omega-3 fatty acids have the potential to alter the course of a number of human diseases, including the physical decline associated with aging.

Supplements for Preventing Osteoporosis

Calcium reduces bone loss and decreases bone turnover. Since calcium is vital to bone building and because the body does not produce calcium naturally, it is therefore imperative that this essential mineral be obtained from food intake and supplements. Numerous studies have shown that calcium supplementation can help decrease bone loss by 30–50 percent.

Vitamin D is needed for the absorption of calcium and mineralization of bone. Evidence supports the use of calcium in combination with vitamin D supplementation, as a preventive treatment of osteoporosis in people aged 50 years or older. Supplementation is best done with vitamin D_3. Stronger bones reduce the risk of bone fractures due to falling, which is a common occurrence in elderly people.

Boron is a trace mineral which, besides maintaining memory and increasing bone cartilage formation, is also vital for the normal growth and health of the body. It helps reduce menopausal symptoms and manages osteoporosis and arthritis naturally. It is believed that boron improves the body's natural ability to absorb calcium and magnesium and activates vitamin D to increase the mineral content in the bones.

Zinc is required to maintain bone mineral density and bone metabolism and is important for your overall mental and physical health.

Copper is an essential trace mineral that is important for bone formation and resorption (bone loss). It is linked with the generation of mesenchymal stem cells that develop osteoblasts in the body, leading to bone development.

Vitamin K$_2$ — Vitamin K, typically known for its role in coagulation, goes way beyond mere blood clotting. In the 1980s, it was discovered that vitamin K helps the body activate and maintain the protein called osteocalcin, which is essential for bone mineralization. Recent research has shown that without vitamin K$_2$, calcium regulation is disrupted.

Manganese is required for the repair of soft bone and tissue and facilitates bone growth and maintenance. It also plays a role in the production of estrogen and progesterone. Manganese is the preferred cofactor of enzymes called glycosyltransferases, which are important for the formation of healthy cartilage and bone. Too much calcium can decrease the absorption of manganese, therefore, the ratio of calcium to manganese supplementation is essential.

5.8 Summary: Maintaining Strong Organ Systems

THE CARDIOVASCULAR SYSTEM

The main interventions to promote heart health are:	
a)	*Exercise*
b)	*Stress Management*
c)	*Supplements*

The main interventions for the vascular system are:	
a)	*Excellent nutrition*
b)	*Exercise*
c)	*Taking correct minerals*
d)	*Maintaining good blood pressure*
e)	*Supplements*

GASTROINTESTINAL SYSTEM

Implementing the 4R program helps rebalance the gastrointestinal tract:	
a)	*Remove — allergens, infections, toxins*
b)	*Replace — gastric acid, digestive enzymes*

c)	Replenish — supplement with healthy probiotics and prebiotics
d)	Repair — provide repairing nutrients, including zinc carnosine for the stomach, glutamine for the small intestine and butyrate for the large intestine.

KIDNEY OR RENAL SYSTEM

a)	Provide enough fluids each day.
b)	Prevent taking chemicals that can damage kidneys — mainly in the form of drugs such as NSAIDs and lithium.
c)	Prevent high sugars in the blood.
d)	Quit smoking.
e)	Maintain a good blood pressure.

LIVER

Below is a list of things you can do to help protect your liver:	
a)	Decrease your sugar intake and refined carbohydrates, as well as bad fats and oils, to prevent the development of fatty liver and liver damage.
b)	Prevent toxins from entering the liver — mainly drugs that are hepatotoxic (NSAIDS) anti inflammatories,

	statins *(unless essential)*, *acetaminophen, and many others.*
c)	*Avoid excess alcohol use to prevent liver damage.*
d)	*Other toxins such as pesticides, heavy metals like mercury from amalgams, excess hormones, xenobiotics, excess iron and copper and PCBs from plastics should also be avoided as much as possible. If these poisons are found in the liver during testing, a full liver detox program, with the assistance of a physician, may need to be carried out.*
e)	*Take supplements that assist liver health.*

NEUROLOGICAL SYSTEM

	Although it may seem that the brain doesn't need a lot of care, the following steps are essential to keep it healthy and functioning well into old age:
a)	*Brain health is very dependent on nutrition. The correct nutrients are required and toxic foods must be removed.*
b)	*Physical exercise plays a major role in brain health.*
c)	*Stimulating your brain is essential. Being creative, solving problems and using your thought processes are*

	essential to stretch the brain and keep it functioning well.
d)	*Remove stress, which can damage the brain.*
e)	*It is important to be productive and busy and not to slip into retirement mode.*
f)	*Keep yourself social and make sure you have daily contact with positive people.*
g)	*Take the appropriate brain supplements.*
h)	*Have purpose and meaning in life.*

MUSCULOSKELETAL SYSTEM

	The muscles and bones form the support system of the body. The deterioration of the bones due to osteoporosis and the weakening of muscles that develop with age can be reversed by doing the following:
a)	*Do appropriate exercises — mainly weight bearing and strength exercises.*
b)	*Work on your posture while sitting and standing.*
c)	*Take the appropriate vitamins, minerals and supplements.*

CHAPTER 6

THE ENDOCRINE SYSTEM

The endocrine system comprises a collection of glands that produce hormones that regulate metabolism, growth and development, tissue function, sexual function, reproduction, sleep and mood, among other things. Included in this system is the thyroid gland, the parathyroid gland, adrenal glands, pancreas, ovaries and testicles. These glands produce hormones which are chemical substances that control and oversee the activity of certain cells or organs. The hormone travels through the blood vessels and each type of hormone attaches to receptors targeted for specific cells or organs, causing a set of reactions to occur in those cells.

For example, the thyroid hormone will attach to receptors on cells, which will cause the cells to metabolize at a more rapid rate and help with weight loss. Adrenaline is a hormone made in the adrenal gland and will attach to heart cells and cause a rapid heartbeat. Insulin attaches to cells which facilitates the transport of glucose from the blood into the cells, in order to metabolize it and produce energy.

Hormones trigger different reactions in the various tissues and organs, and it is therefore essential to keep a good balance of hormone function so that they all work in harmony to maintain the effective functioning of the body.

As we age, the efficiency and levels of our hormones change and should be regulated accordingly. The following are the main hormones that affect body functioning.

6.1 Thyroid

The thyroid gland is a small butterfly-shaped organ that is

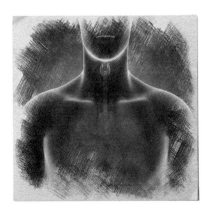

situated at the base of the neck above the chest. Hormones produced in the thyroid regulate almost every cell in the human body by controlling the amount of oxygen cells use, and the rate at which organs and cells convert nutrients into energy. The thyroid gland works in conjunction with the pituitary gland, which controls the amount of hormones released by the thyroid.

One of the main causes of thyroid dysfunction is a lack of a constant iodine supply, which is needed to produce the thyroid hormone. Illnesses as a result of very high or very low levels of thyroid hormones can wreak havoc on the body. Autoimmune thyroid disease occurs when antibodies attack the thyroid, resulting in either an overproduction or underproduction of the thyroid hormone.

When you have hyperthyroidism, your body produces excessive amounts of T3 and T4, which are associated with the regulation of your metabolism. High levels mean a high metabolism, which speeds up some of your body's processes. It is associated with the following symptoms, although not all of them may be experienced:

❑ Change in appetite — either an increase or decrease
❑ Fatigue
❑ Difficulty sleeping
❑ Muscle weakness
❑ Heat intolerance
❑ Heart palpitations
❑ Shortness of breath
❑ Problems with fertility
❑ Thinning of hair, which can also become brittle
❑ Nervousness, anxiety and irritability
❑ Changes in menstrual patterns
❑ Sweating

Hypothyroidism occurs when there is an underproduction of T3 and T4 cells. These symptoms are as follows:

❑ Fatigue
❑ Weakness
❑ Weight gain
❑ Coarse, dry hair and hair loss
❑ Intolerance to cold temperatures
❑ Frequent muscle cramps and aches
❑ Depression and irritability
❑ Menstrual irregularity

❑ Memory loss
❑ Decreased libido

It is important to check your thyroid and thyroid antibody levels by means of a blood test. Any imbalance must be addressed by your physician or functional medicine provider.

Two common conditions that do not necessarily require medical treatment are hypothyroidism (low thyroid) due to either iodine deficiency or an autoimmune condition called Hashimoto's disease. Hashimoto's has high thyroid antibodies, which damages the thyroid and is often associated with gluten sensitivity or celiac disease. One may find that cutting out gluten from one's diet may lead to an improvement in this condition. If there are no antibodies, one can measure for iodine deficiency or even try iodine replacement by consulting a practitioner in functional medicine. If thyroid hormone replacement is required, one may benefit from replacing T3 and T4, and again a functional medicine practitioner would know how to prescribe this.

6.2 Adrenal Hormones

The adrenal glands are two glands that sit above both kidneys. They are divided into two distinct parts — the outer part is called the adrenal cortex and the inner part is the adrenal medulla. They are both necessary for secreting hormones, however, the adrenal cortex produces hormones that are essential for our existence and the medulla produces hormones that are non-essential to life.

The adrenal cortex produces three hormones:

1. **Aldosterone** helps maintain the body's salt and water levels, which in turn regulates blood pressure. Without aldosterone, the kidney loses excessive amounts of salt and water, leading to severe dehydration and low blood pressure.
2. **Cortisol** helps balance the effects of insulin in breaking down sugar for energy and regulates the metabolism of fats, protein and carbohydrates. It also works together with corticosterone to regulate the immune response and suppress inflammation in the body.
3. **Adrenal androgens** are hormones that play a role in the production of testosterone and estrogen in the body.

The adrenal medulla produces adrenaline (epinephrine) and noradrenaline (norepinephrine), which are the first responders to acute stress or the fight-or-flight response.

There are illnesses that require medical treatment, as in the case of Cushing's syndrome where cortisol levels are very high, and Addison's syndrome, which is an autoimmune disease resulting from the failure to produce sufficient cortisol and cortisol levels are very low.

If a medical reason for adrenal dysfunction has been ruled out, then chronic stress is a common cause for adrenal dysfunction. Initially, high levels of cortisol occur. After some time, the brain, which is adversely affected by this high cortisol, will send a feedback message to the adrenals to shut down production, resulting in low cortisol levels and causing the body to "crash." This syndrome is called adrenal fatigue. It needs to be managed by reducing stress and taking appropriate supplements to either reduce cortisol or boost cortisol production, depending on the levels. An accurate way to test cortisol is either with a salivary test or a urine test.

Symptoms of adrenal fatigue include:

- Difficulty getting up in the morning and fatigue throughout the day
- Body aches
- Unexplained weight loss
- Low blood pressure
- Lightheadedness
- Loss of body hair
- Skin discoloration (hyperpigmentation)
- Cravings for salty food
- Weak immune system
- Inability to handle stressful situations

In my experience in my family practice, I have had many patients who have presented with fatigue, irritability, anger, weakness or many of the symptoms mentioned above. Full panels of the typical testing were done and often no abnormalities detected, until I discovered that one needs to take a full lifestyle history and see how the patient is coping in life. An important test that needs to be taken is one that measures your cortisol levels, preferably in the saliva 4 times during the day. With this additional information, I frequently discovered that all these symptoms were due to adrenal fatigue and needed a full program to treat their adrenals. Naturally, great results were achieved.

6.3 Pancreas

The pancreas is an endocrine gland that produces several important hormones, including insulin and glucagon, which circulate in the blood. These are associated with the control of blood sugar levels and metabolism in the body. The 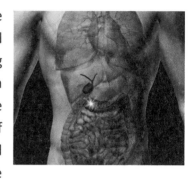 pancreas is also a digestive organ which secretes pancreatic juice to help neutralize acidity from the partially digested food that moves from the stomach, as well as digestive enzymes that expedite digestion and absorption of nutrients in the small intestine.

Insulin and glucagon are both secreted by the islet cells in the pancreas to help regulate blood sugar levels, but they work in a contradicting manner. As the blood glucose levels increase, the pancreas secretes more and more insulin to counteract it. When the blood glucose levels decrease, insulin reduction follows suit. Insulin affects a number of cells, including muscle, red blood cells and fat cells which absorb glucose out of the blood, thereby lowering high blood sugar levels. Glucagon works in the opposite manner — when blood sugar levels are very low, glucagon is secreted to counteract this effect.

It is therefore essential that the correct insulin levels are maintained in the body. Insufficient insulin production or a damaged pancreas can lead to diabetes. Type 1 diabetes is due to an autoimmune reaction that damages the pancreas and causes low and then absent insulin levels.

If the cell receptors which react to insulin become less sensitive or resistant to insulin, then more and more insulin is produced to retain the correct glucose levels. This is known as insulin resistance and is mainly due to eating a poor diet, being overweight and having excess adipose or fat cells in the body. The excess demand for insulin will eventually cause the beta cells that produce insulin to wear out and this leads to the development of type 2 diabetes.

The following medical conditions are associated with insulin resistance:

- Type 2 diabetes
- Arteriosclerosis
- Fatty liver disease
- Skin lesions and tags

Insulin resistance can be controlled if attention is paid to your diet, exercise routine and weight control. Our supplement Resulin™ contains Chromium Picolinate, Berberine, Bitter Melon Extract and Alpha Lipoic Acid, which all assist with insulin sensitivity.

6.4 Sex Hormones

For Males

Testosterone is the hormone in males that is responsible for the deep voice, facial and body hair and muscle mass. As we age, the level of testosterone slowly diminishes leading to a menopause-like state known as andropause. It is a much more subtle phase, and sometimes goes unnoticed by men, although it is estimated that 10% of testosterone is lost per decade in men over the age of 30.

There are two main functions of testosterone: androgenic, which includes the growth, development and maintenance of the male reproductive tract, and anabolic effects, which include growth of muscle strength and mass, increased bone density and strength, and the growth of body hair. Testosterone also affects other systems, such as the brain and heart, as well as stimulating red blood cell production in the bone marrow.

The signs and symptoms of testosterone deficiency are:

- Erectile dysfunction
- Reduced libido
- Depression or sadness
- Reduced muscle mass
- Increased body fat
- Decreased motivation
- Gynecomastia or breast development
- Hot flashes
- Reduced brain reaction time

Testosterone levels are checked by means of a blood test. Low levels can be raised with testosterone replacement therapy, but caution must be exercised in young males and males who want to remain fertile. There are a number of different ways of receiving the treatments, including injections that provide long-acting testosterone, skin patches and gels or pellets that are inserted under the skin. Before resorting to medicinal testosterone replacement, natural methods should be tried first to boost your levels. These include regular exercise — particularly strength exercises, stress management techniques and taking certain nutraceuticals. It is important to measure testosterone levels and to speak to a doctor qualified in functional or anti-aging medicine to manage a deficiency.

Estrogen hormones also play an important role in males. As teenagers, men have high testosterone levels and low estrogen levels. As men age, testosterone begins to convert to estrogen due to the aromatase reaction. Aromatase is found most prevalently in fat cells, especially around the waist, which means the more body fat a man has, the higher the estrogen levels will be. Excess alcohol and zinc deficiency are added instigators in the aromatase reaction. High estrogen levels in men contribute to heart disease, gynecomastia (enlarged breasts) as well as prostate cancer. A lack of estrogen or estrogen receptors in males can cause osteoporosis, glucose intolerance and abnormal lipid profiles. Therefore, a healthy balance of estrogen and testosterone must be maintained.

DHEA is a hormone produced mainly in the adrenal gland. Production peaks at age 20 and then starts to decline. Although DHEA is a precursor to testosterone, it has not been proven that taking DHEA supplements boost testosterone levels. DHEA however, may have some positive effects, including benefiting the cardiovascular system and improving brain function and metabolic syndrome. If you have low levels, it is important to speak to your doctor about DHEA replacement.

For Females

The female hormones, which are mainly estrogen and progesterone, control the development and regulation of the female reproductive system, the menstrual cycle and the ability to become pregnant. With age, hormone levels decline, usually with progesterone leading the way until the menstrual cycle ceases completely and menopause sets in. Estrogen and progesterone have important roles to play for many systems in females.

Estrogen: Estrogen hormones are responsible for the growth and development of female characteristics as well as reproduction. It is produced primarily in the ovaries before menopause and in small amounts in other tissue after menopause. There are three types of estrogen: estrone E1 and estradiol E2, which are produced in the ovaries in premenopausal women, and estriol E3, which is produced in the placenta during pregnancy. Estradiol is the predominant estrogen during the reproductive years, estrone is the predominant circulating estrogen during menopause and estriol is predominant during pregnancy. All forms of estrogen are synthesized from androgens, especially testosterone and androstenedione, by the enzyme aromatase.

Estrogen plays a number of roles in the female body. They are as follows:

1. During the reproductive years, each month when an egg follicle is released, estrogen thickens the uterus lining to prepare it for pregnancy.
2. Estrogen works together with calcium, vitamin D and other hormones and minerals to build strong bones. After the age of 30, the body breaks down more bone than it makes and if this process is not curbed and reversed, osteoporosis develops.
3. Estrogen maintains the thickness and mucous production of cells in the vaginal walls, preventing them from becoming thin and dry. It also prevents the urethra, which carries urine from the bladder to the outside of the body, from thinning, which can cause urinary tract infections.
4. Estrogen influences our physical and emotional state and can cause breast tenderness, hot flashes, irregular menstrual periods, irritability and mood swings.

Estrogen levels usually decrease with age, as you approach menopause or perimenopause. There are a number of symptoms that indicate the change in estrogen levels, including:

- Reduction or change in menstrual cycles

- Vaginal dryness and painful intercourse
- Increased yeast and UTI infections
- Emotional changes such as mood swings, depression and irritability
- Forgetfulness, brain fog and poor concentration
- Sleep issues and fatigue
- Weight gain
- Headaches and migraines
- Decreased libido

There are 2 types of estrogen receptors on the cells: alpha and beta receptors. Alpha receptors are predominant in breast, uterine and ovarian tissue, and when stimulated, will cause cell division and may have a pro-cancer affect. Estrone E1 has strong alpha receptor effects and should not be taken, particularly after menopause. Beta receptors occur in the brain, bone, intestinal lining and prostate and when stimulated by estrogen, will have a positive effect on these tissues. Estradiol E2 effects both alpha and beta receptors and estriol E3 has a stronger beta receptor effect, and these two types of estrogen are the preferable choice after menopause. This avoids the dangerous effects of stimulated cell division and provides the positive effects required after menopause.

Hormone replacement therapy has been selected for the treatment of menopausal symptoms including hot flashes, night sweats, mood swings, memory loss, weight gain, sleep issues and sexual dysfunction. It has also been indicated in the positive effects it has on diabetes, cataracts and the hydration and elasticity of the skin and preventing osteoporosis. Nowadays, bioidentical hormones are the preferred choice, as they are man-made hormones derived from plant estrogens that are identical to the estrogen in human beings. It is important to use a health practitioner experienced in hormone replacement therapy to help you select the correct treatment for you.

Progesterone: Prior to menopause, progesterone is produced during the second half of the menstrual cycle by the ovaries. Progesterone causes the endometrium to secret special proteins that help prepare it for the reception and nourishment of a fertilized egg. If the egg does not become fertilized, the endometrium lining falls away during a menstrual cycle, and the production of progesterone drops. Pregnancy occurs when the egg becomes fertilized. Progesterone is then produced in large amounts in the placenta, which helps encourage the growth of glands in the breast for milk production. Progesterone also plays an important role in the development of the fetus and strengthens the pelvic wall muscles in preparation for labor. The level of progesterone continues to increase throughout the pregnancy until after the birth.

Correct levels of progesterone are vital during a woman's reproductive years. Low levels can have the following effects:

1. Trouble becoming pregnant or staying pregnant
2. Abnormal uterine bleeding
3. Headaches and migraines
4. Mood swings and irritability

5. Low libido
6. Hot flashes
7. Irregular menstrual cycles
8. Bloating
9. Joint pains

Progesterone has many effects in the body, and it is essential to balance the levels with estrogen. If hormone replacement therapy is required, make sure you take bioidentical hormones that are identical to human progesterone, as opposed to progestin, which is a chemical similar to progesterone but has many negative effects. The benefits of taking bioidentical hormones (BHRT) are that they are safer than synthetic hormones, they have fewer side effects and are made from natural substances. Other benefits include the prevention of osteoporosis and improved concentration.

Testosterone: Testosterone is usually seen as a male hormone. But that is not the case. Testosterone is produced in the adrenal glands and the ovaries even after menopause, and women who have their ovaries removed will experience low testosterone levels and the symptoms that accompany it.

Testosterone performs a number of functions in the woman's body, including:

- Maintaining muscle strength and lean muscle mass
- It is vital for bone strength
- Improves your overall well-being and energy levels
- Brain function

- It affects libido

Symptoms of low testosterone are as follows:

- Low sexual drive and satisfaction
- Lethargy
- Muscle weakness
- Depression

On the flip side of the scale, testosterone can occur in excess in premenopausal women, which is referred to as PCOS, or polycystic ovarian syndrome. This illness causes fluid-filled clusters of pearl-sized cysts to develop in the ovaries, and can result in the following symptoms:

- Irregular, heavy or non-existent menstrual cycle
- Infertility
- Excess or unwanted facial or body hair growth
- Thinning hair on the scalp
- Weight problems, including weight gain around the waist
- Skin problems, including skin tags, darkening skin and acne
- Anxiety or depression

Testosterone can either be converted to estrogen by the aromatase enzyme or to dihydrotestosterone (DHT) by the alpha reductase enzyme. Too much DHT can cause hair loss in women, excess facial and body hair and acne. There are natural ways to reduce DHT production, including certain herbs and supplements, exercising, getting enough sleep, keeping stress levels down and following a healthy diet.

Hormone replacement therapy is another option, but should be discussed with your healthcare practitioner first.

Maintaining a balance of your hormones is important even after menopause, and the diagnosis and treatment of menopause should be discussed with a health provider qualified in the field of bioidentical hormone replacement.

CHAPTER 7

AN OVERVIEW OF HOW THE LIFE PROTOCOL WORKS TOGETHER

The fundamental goal of our anti-aging program is to ensure healthy, functioning cells in all the tissues and preserve the DNA material for cell replication and the mitochondria for energy production. Being young and aging are really defined by the health and youthfulness of our cells in all the tissues. So, what influences the body at a cellular level?

L — Lifestyle

External influences that affect all segments of your health include:

- Healthy nutrition
- Fitness
- Stress management
- Avoiding toxins

These all provide the basic underlying foundation that influence how the body functions. If you do not receive the correct healthy building blocks that the body needs, then optimal functioning can never be achieved. The external fuel for enabling the body to work and for maintaining it must be of high quality and non-toxic.

There are a number of barriers lining all the major structures that transport and absorb these nutrients into the tissue and around the body. These barriers are made up of a single layer of cells which allow certain substances to enter, whilst keeping others out.

The three main barriers are:

1. **The epithelial layer** — This a single layer of cells in the gut that determines which nutrients and/or toxins are absorbed into the body. If this layer is damaged, then a leaky gut develops and many damaging substances can enter the body.
2. The **endothelium** is a single layer of cells lining the inner layer of the blood vessels. If this lining is damaged, plaque will begin to build up inside the arteries, which could lead to a heart attack or stroke.
3. The **blood-brain barrier** is a layer of cells that protects and selects what enters the brain. This layer of cells must remain intact to avoid damage to the brain cells.

All these barriers will function well provided the following four criteria are met:

1. There is no inflammation or allergies that can cause damage.
2. There are no toxins present.
3. There is no abnormal immune reaction that can cause damage.

4. There is an adequate supply of healthy nutrients, vitamins and minerals.

Therefore, in order to maintain healthy barriers and ensure optimal absorption, it is imperative that we take the correct nutrients.

In addition to providing healthy external factors to the cells, we then have to make sure that the major internal influences on the cells are efficient and balanced. Cells and tissue are affected by the immune system, that can either protect or damage them. Hormones attach to receptors on cells and influence cell function, which is why it is important to ensure that the endocrine system is in balance. The nervous system also affects many different organs in the body and must function in a parasympathetic rest-and-digest mode, as opposed to the fight-or-flight mode.

I — Immune

The next layer of protection is to maintain a well functioning immune system. The immune system prevents infections and is vital to kill the early onset of cancer cells. It is important to boost a weak immune system with the correct nutrients, vitamins and herbs, as well as stress reduction.

However, we do not want an overstimulated immune system, which can be brought about by either introducing allergens into the system that can cause an allergic reaction, such as allergies to foods, or a stronger auto-immune response initiated by toxins entering the body. This excess immune activity will cause damage.

E — Endocrine

The E which comes after F in life, really fits in now. E represents the endocrine system, which in fact has a controlling affect over the entire body. The hormones produced by various glands are transported to all the different cells in the body and help maintain the efficient functioning of many of the organs and tissues. The endocrine system must be kept well balanced and productive.

F — Functional System

The functional system embodies all the main organ systems that play a crucial role in keeping optimal functioning within the body:

- The heart and lungs distribute oxygen to the tissue, and the blood vessels provide nutrients.
- The gut digests and absorbs nutrients and removes waste.
- The liver and kidneys filter and remove toxins and waste products.
- The brain and nervous system control and assimilate information and influence the reactions in the body.

When any one of these systems begins to display signs of fatigue or illness, it is an indication that all or parts of the main influences are not working well.

The overall aim for all these systems is to maintain healthy cells in all the tissues. Providing healthy nutrients, balanced hormones, a normal immune response, a relaxed nerve function and the removal of toxins will ensure efficient, youthful cells and prevent the acceleration of aging at the cellular level.

The master influences are

- lifestyle factors;
- the immune and inflammatory responses;
- hormone balance;
- the nervous system.

We see the body as a unified machine that works as one unit, and essentially the same factors affect each and every part. By keeping the major influencers in good shape, their impact will trickle down to all the cells and enable the body to continue to work in harmony, thereby preserving youthfulness. This is the basis of our anti-aging program.

CHAPTER 8

SUPPLEMENTS FOR EACH SYSTEM AND EACH PATHWAY TO SLOW AGING

SCIENTIFIC

The LIFE protocol is based on scientific analysis and an abundance of research that has proven results and positively works. All the components that have been included in the program have proven scientific evidence that they prevent disease and improve life and vitality. These factors have a much more powerful effect than drugs.

Time limitations, pressure and even laziness may cause us to slip into an unhealthy groove, and it is definitely much easier continuing along with an unhealthy lifestyle as opposed to slowing down and taking the time and making the effort to make some crucial lifestyle changes. It is easy to obtain and take prescription medication for high cholesterol or high blood pressure rather than getting a prescription for the above lifestyle changes and additional natural supplements. The latter option is far more beneficial and will provide much broader and long-term benefits.

All our recommended supplements have been carefully formulated to achieve the desired effects, based on scientific evidence that they work. The synergy between taking the correct supplements and making the correct lifestyle changes will have a powerful outcome on your overall health.

COMPREHENSIVE AND INDIVIDUALIZED

Although eating a balanced diet and enjoying a little sunshine definitely helps the body get some vitamins, not enough is obtained in this manner. It is therefore important to cover all bases with vitamin and mineral supplements that assist with strengthening the body. Supplements can be for general strengthening or be system specific, and it is important to obtain an individualized prescription that covers all your health issues. Taking multivitamins and supplements is not ideal, as it does not target specific issues that you may have. It is best to look at your overall health picture and treat it accordingly. The Beyoung Health Quiz will highlight your needs and areas that require special attention.

SYNERGISTIC

When taking a few different supplements, it is important to ensure that they work in harmony with one another. At Beyoung Clinics, our supplements are very system specific, targeting and assisting distinct organs. It is important to manage a range of vitamins when taking them together — to avoid the problem of taking too high a dose of a specific ingredient. There is a daily recommended dosage for each vitamin, and if two supplements are taken together that both have the same vitamin contained in them, for example vitamin D, the total of both supplements should be within the daily dosage range. Therefore, a synergistic effect must be established, and the vitamin dosage must mesh when various supplements are taken together.

SUMMARY OF SUPPLEMENTS FOR INDIVIDUAL NEEDS

Vitamins are not only formulated for individuals with existing health issues, but the correct supplements should be taken by everyone as a preventative for developing illnesses.

Ignite supplements are our own range of vitamins that cover an assortment of systems in the body. They are as follows:

RESPARK™

RESPARK™ has been formulated with the most effective and purest of natural ingredients to help strengthen and support overall bodily function and maintenance as you age. It is designed to specifically replace all the vitamins and minerals that decline with age and is appropriate for everyone.

It contains Curcumin, Magnesium, Vitamin C, Lycopene, Zinc Picolinate, Vitamin K_2, Vitamin B_1 B_2 B_3 B_6 B_{12} D_3, Beta Carotene, Copper Citrate, Methylselenocysteine and Marine AlgaeCal, which is a natural calcium with minerals derived from special algae.

REKINDLE™

REKINDLE™ is a supplement uniquely formulated to incorporate ingredients shown to slow down the aging process. It works directly on the energy production ability, efficiency and lifespan of the mitochondria in cells, while at the same time repairing damage caused by oxidation. It contains Resveratrol, Pterostilbene, L-Carnosine, CoQ10 and Astaxanthin.

RESULIN™

RESULIN™ was formulated to help demote insulin resistance and promote healthy blood sugar levels. This supplement is recommended for individuals with marginally elevated glucose and Hba1c levels. It combines the top natural scientifically proven ingredients to maintain a healthy blood sugar balance, including Chromium, Berberine, Bitter Melon Extract and Alpha Lipoic Acid.

REFLOW™

REFLOW™ supplements are uniquely formulated to help strengthen and support vascular health. Maintaining a healthy vascular system is imperative for the prevention of heart disease and other diseases associated with aging. It includes Pomegranate Extract, Pine Bark Extract, Grapeseed Extract and Olive Leaf Extract.

RENEURO™

RENEURO™ has been formulated with ingredients that have been scientifically proven to help enhance memory and prevent memory loss. This supplement helps promote mental clarity, learning abilities, memory, intelligence and improve your mood. Ingredients include Bacopa Monnieri Extract, Magnesium Threonate, Fisetin and Lion's Mane Extract.

RESTEROL™

RESTEROL™ has been uniquely formulated to help promote a healthy lipid profile and cholesterol levels. Maintaining lower levels of cholesterol helps reduce, slow-down or even stop the buildup of plaque in the arteries, which can increase the risk of heart disease. It contains Tocotrienols (a form of vitamin E), Pantethine and Citrus Bergamot Extract.

REWAKE™

REWAKE™ has been uniquely formulated to help energize and rejuvenate. The main objective of this product is to promote healthy cortisol levels, which affect the body's stress response and metabolism mechanism. The herbs and nutrients in REWAKE™ are known to eliminate fatigue by revitalizing the adrenal glands through balancing the hormones it produces. Our supplement contains Vitamin C, B_2, B_6, Ashwagandha and Rhodiola Root Extract.

REMOBILIZE™

REMOBILIZE™ has been scientifically formulated to help promote a healthy inflammatory response through the inhibition of inflammation pathways. The nutrients contained in this supplement also help reduce pain due to inflammation, and include Curcumin, Boswellia and PPQ (Pyrroloquinoline Quinone Disodium).

REGLOW™

REGLOW™ has been uniquely formulated to help you look younger and healthier, by stimulating increased collagen production and elasticity in the skin. This helps dull the appearance of fine lines and wrinkles, while locking in moisture. The supplement includes Lipowheat, Polypodium Leucotomos, Beta Carotene, Vitamin C, Green Tea Extract and Hyaluronic Acid.

REBONE™

REBONE™ has been specially formulated with vitamins and minerals that are crucial for bone-building and overall bone health. It is critical to build strong, dense bones whilst you are young and keeping them strong and healthy as you age. The nutraceutical contains AlgaeCal (calcium and magnesium obtained from special algae), Zinc Picolinate, Manganese Bisglycinate, Boron Citrate, Copper II Citrate, Vitamin K_2 (menaquinone-7) and Vitamin D_3 (Calciferol).

RESERENE™

RESERENE™ contains essential nutrients, vitamins and herbs that promote tranquility while helping to calm anxiety. Being able to stay calm and maintain a healthy sleep regimen under duress enables our brain and body to recover and rejuvenate. The nutraceutical contains Passion Flower, Inositol, Lemon Balm and L-Theanine and taken together with the core anti-aging supplements RESPARK™ and REKINDLE™, RESERENE™ promotes healthy aging.

RELINE™

RELINE™ is a supplement that promotes gut and intestine health, by supporting a healthy gastric lining, calming indigestion and discouraging the formation of ulcers. It contains Zinc L-Carnosine, Marshmallow Root, Slippery Elm, Mastic Gum Powder and Gastro Enzyme Blend.

CHAPTER 9

ATTITUDE: AGING, THE BEGINNING OF A NEW LIFE

I have worked with many thousands of people, and during that time I have seen amazing trends. The way people shift into the aging role becomes quite obvious when one observes their attitude and appearance as they slip past 50 and into their 60s and older.

There are two distinct groups that people fit into. The first are those individuals who do not notice or feel their age and remain fully engaged and active. They remain fit and mobile and lead a busy lifestyle. These people are not programmed to see aging as a slowing down time and a time to prepare for old age, but rather they continue to live each day to the fullest, and do not view themselves as being old. The second group are those that fit into the aging process. They slow down, do less, their posture is stooped with their head held forward, they lose muscle strength and they become frail and accepting that this is part of the normal aging process.

Attitude is the essential difference! The first group has an attitude that "now is the time to make the most of life" — delving into new jobs and hobbies, keeping fit and strong and remaining engaged in all aspects of life. They enjoy sharing their wisdom that has accumulated with age and socializing with friends and family.

On the other hand, the built-in program of working hard in order to retire and then being careful to take things easy, and of course only using one's brain in passive activities and being nervous about overexerting oneself, is all part of living the script of becoming old. Our approach is to be 50 at 70 and 60 at 80, so that we do not live the life of an old person, but rather think young and act young.

CHAPTER 10

BREAK LIMITATIONS AND BOUNDARIES

So where do we set our targets?

- Do we start an old man's or old girl's exercise program by walking twice around the block and doing some light weights and a tai chi class once a week?
- Or do we join a gym and get a trainer for a while to get us started and do serious weight training and really build our atrophied muscles?
- Do we start interval training and build our fitness so that we can really sprint on the treadmill with intervals?
- Do we spend more time watching T.V. or doing the same old shopping every day?
- Do we read the same news each day or do we start the small business that we have always dreamed of doing?
- Do we decide to learn a new language or sign up to do a course at college that really interests us?

We can accelerate aging by settling into the role of retirement and getting old, or we can ignore this inevitable stage and do all the things that we have always wanted to do with energy and vigor — and not be limited by our age.

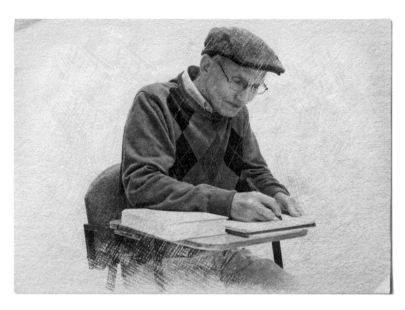

Obviously, you will not be able to bench press what you did at 30 years old, but you can do much more than you think if you are not limited by your perceived limitations.

CHAPTER 11

BEYOUNG'S PROGRAM IN A NUTSHELL

11.1 GET A BASELINE CHECK UP

Undergo a battery of screening tests necessary to prevent the onset of serious illness. Visit your physician and ensure that all tests are done according to your age, family history and personal risks. These can be life saving. Once this has been done, you can move onto regaining your youth.

11.2 TAKE ON THE CORE ANTI-AGING STEPS

Improve cellular and mitochondrial function by incorporating the changes below:

• Nutritional adjustments
• Exercise routine (avoid over exercising)
• Stress management
• Sufficient sleep
• Avoid toxins
• Prevent telomere shortening

- ◆ Take sufficient vitamin D in order to get good blood levels of vitamin D

- ◆ Take Astaxanthin — this is a potent antioxidant, which has anti-inflammatory and DNA protective properties

- ◆ Take Coenzyme Q10 — this is an enzyme used by every cell in the body. CoQ10 is not only necessary for producing cellular energy, but also for defending cells from damage caused by harmful free radicals. It helps neutralize the harmful free radicals and protects the DNA in cells from oxidative stress that causes the effects of aging.

- ◆ Take magnesium

- ◆ Take vitamin B12 in order to get sufficient levels of vitamin B12

- ◆ Take vitamin A

- ◆ Resveratrol and pterostilbene

→ **All the above vitamins can be taken together in our two Ignite supplements called**
  - ◆ *Respark™ and*
  - ◆ *Rekindle™*

→ Prevent inflammation — Follow an anti-inflammatory diet to reduce inflammation. Ensure that you keep your stress levels to a minimum and take supplements that include curcumin and boswellia.

→ Balance your hormones — Consult with an anti-aging or functional medicine doctor who will test your hormone levels and draw up a hormone profile for you. Discuss the possible use of bioidentical hormones.

11.3 GET A LIFEPRINT

It is helpful to obtain a good understanding of your strengths and weaknesses in order to build up areas in which you are lacking. For a comprehensive profile, join our Beyoung Clinic program. We will give you an in-depth understanding about your health and provide you with full support and follow-up appointments to implement an anti-aging solution and help you make life-changing decisions that will impact your life.

It is crucial to understand your personal lifeprint. This will clarify which areas of your health have the potential for becoming problematic down the line. You can then focus on those systems that need preventive action to delay and even prevent the onset of real problems.

Here is an example plan:

Step 1 — Visit your local physician and request the appropriate screening tests for your age. Make sure that you do all these tests as they may be life saving.

Step 2 — Review your current lifestyle choices to ensure they are optimal for good health. This includes:

- *Nutrition* — Start a healthy nutrition program. Beyoung has an excellent nutrition plan that is easy to implement and follow, and if you have specific risk areas, for example a potential for dementia, prediabetes or high inflammation, our plan can be adjusted to accommodate these health issues accordingly. If this seems overwhelming, a nutrition coach can help guide you to put your program in place.

- *Exercise* — Make sure you have a good exercise routine tailor-made for you. It is important to cover the exercises recommended in the fitness section. If you cannot implement a suitable, enjoyable and sustainable program on your own, it is essential to seek the guidance of a fitness coach to set one up for you and to monitor your progress.

- *Sleep* — Get the optimal sleep that your body needs.

- *Stress* — Minimize your stress levels. Do not underestimate this area. It may be the most important intervention that you can take on. Read my book *The Heart of the Matter*, which gives practical tips on how to manage your stress. If necessary, seek professional guidance.

Step 3 — Get your LIFEPRINT. This may show weaknesses in your cardiovascular health, or bone and muscle health. Any areas that are weak need to be strengthened by implementing the appropriate lifestyle changes above and by taking the appropriate supplements.

APPENDIX

9 Steps

TIPS FOR HEALTHY FOOD SHOPPING

The first step to good nutrition is to make the right choices, beginning with your shopping. If you have the right ingredients in your home, you will automatically eat and prepare healthier foods. When you go food shopping, focus on the perimeter of the store where the fresh produce and perishables are usually located. It is also important to read the labels on packaged foods to determine what ingredients are contained therein.

STEP 01

PRODUCE

Always buy a selection of fresh fruit and vegetables to snack on and include in your meals. Carrots, celery, cucumbers, peppers, kolrabi and cauliflower, as well as apples, pears and clementinas are always good to keep in the kitchen.

STEP 02

FROZEN VEGETABLES

Keep a supply of frozen vegetables on hand for back-up meals or preparing something in a hurry. They can be added to soups, sauces, rices or quick dishes.

STEP 03

NUTS AND SEEDS

Buy raw nuts and seeds such as almonds, cashews, walnuts, pumpkin and sunflower seeds. Add them to cereal, fruits and side dishes.

STEP 04

OLIVE OIL

Purchase and use extra virgin olive oil and coconut oil for salads and side dishes. Cook with coconut oil.

STEP 05

DAIRY PRODUCTS

Buy healthy dairy products including cottage cheese and yogurt and avoid milk and yellow cheese. Non dairy alternatives such as almond, rice and soy milks are a good option.

STEP 06

WHOLE GRAIN BREADS AND PASTAS

Purchase whole wheat pasta, brown rice, bulgar, oats, quineoa and millet, as well as whole grain cereals like puffed and shredded wheat and other whole grain products.

STEP 07

PROTEIN

Buy lean, fresh meat, poultry and fish for grilling, roasting and sauteing.

STEP 08

EAT BEFORE YOU SHOP

Never shop on an empty stomach - this will cause you to buy unnecessary items that are usually unhealthy and packed with sugar.

STEP 09

SKIP THE SNACK ISLE

It is preferrable to shop with a list. If not, make sure you skip the isles with snack foods, cookies, cakes, candies and sodas. They are high in unhealthy fats, sugar and calories and tempt the hungry shopper.

Food Reference Table

GREEN FOODS	YELLOW FOODS	RED FOODS
THIS IS THE BASIS FOR YOUR DIET AND SHOULD BE EATEN DAILY OR AT LEAST TWICE WEEKLY	THESE FOODS SHOULD BE EATEN SPARINGLY, INTERSPERSED WITH THE GREEN FOOD LIST	THESE FOODS SHOULD BE AVOIDED ALTOGETHER IF POSSIBLE.
Nuts	Meat (grass fed)	Candies / Chocolate
Fish (wild, not farmed)	Chicken (free range)	Baked goods
Berries	Eggs (free range)	Fried Foods
Pomegranate	Cheese	Sweetened Condiments
Sprouts	Fish	Salad Dressings with sugar
Orange / Red Vegetables	Corn	Iced Coffee
Cruciferous Vegetables	Granola Bars	Pasta
Beans	Rice Cakes	Potatoes
Legumes	Sushi	Unhealthy Oils
Vegetable Soup	Tofu	Sweetened Fruit Juice
Seeds	Veggie Burgers	Soda
Green Tea	Rice	
Green Leafy Vegetables	Wine	
Healthy Fruits		
Whole Grains		
Olive Oil		
Avocado		
Filtered Water		

A. General supplements recommended for everyone

RESPARK™

RESPARK™ has been formulated with the most effective and purest of natural ingredients to help strengthen and support overall bodily function and maintenance as you age. It is designed to specifically replace all the vitamins and minerals that decline with age and is useful for everyone. It contains Curcumin, Magnesium, Vitamin C, Lycopene, Zinc Picolinate, Vitamin K_2, Vitamin B_1 B_2 B_3 B_6 B_{12} D_3, Beta Carotene, Copper Citrate, Methylselenocysteine and Marine AlgaeCal, which is a natural calcium derived from special algae.

REKINDLE™

REKINDLE™ is a supplement uniquely formulated to incorporate ingredients shown to slow down the aging process and that works directly on the energy production ability, efficiency and lifespan of the mitochondria in cells, while at the same time repairing damage caused by oxidation. It contains Resveratrol, Pterostilbene, L-Carnosine, CoQ10 and Astaxanthin.

The following vitamins are system-specific and should be taken with a doctor's prior consent:

RESULIN™

RESULIN™ was formulated to help demote insulin resistance and promote healthy blood sugar levels. This supplement is recommended for individuals with marginally elevated glucose and Hba1c levels. It combines the top natural scientifically proven ingredients to maintain a healthy blood sugar balance, including Chromium, Berberine, Bitter Melon Extract and Alpha Lipoic Acid.

REFLOW™

REFLOW™ supplements are uniquely formulated to help strengthen and support vascular health. Maintaining a healthy vascular system is imperative for the prevention of heart disease and other diseases associated with aging. It includes Pomegranate Extract, Pine Bark Extract, Grapeseed Extract and Olive Leaf Extract.

RENEURO™

RENEURO™ has been formulated with ingredients that have been scientifically proven to help enhance memory and prevent memory loss. This supplement helps promote mental clarity, learning abilities, memory, intelligence and improve your mood. Ingredients include, Bacopa Monnieri Extract, Magnesium Threonate, Fisetin and Lion's Mane Extract.

RESTEROL™

RESTEROL™ has been uniquely formulated to help promote a healthy lipid profile and cholesterol levels. Maintaining lower levels of cholesterol helps reduce, slow-down or even stop the buildup of plaque in the arteries, which can increase the risk of heart disease. It contains Tocotrienols (a form of vitamin E), Pantethine and Citrus Bergamot Extract.

REWAKE™

REWAKE™ has been uniquely formulated to help energize and rejuvenate. The main objective of this product is to promote healthy cortisol levels, which affect the body's stress response and metabolism mechanism. The herbs and nutrients in REWAKE™ are known to eliminate fatigue by revitalizing the adrenal glands through balancing the hormones it produces. Our supplement contains Vitamin C, B_2, B_6, Ashwagandha and Rhodiola Root Extract.

REMOBILIZE™

REMOBILIZE™ has been scientifically formulated to help promote a healthy inflammatory response through the inhibition of inflammation pathways. The nutrients contained in this supplement also help reduce pain due to inflammation, and include Curcumin, Boswellia and PPQ (Pyrroloquinoline Quinone Disodium).

REGLOW™

REGLOW™ has been uniquely formulated to help you look younger and healthier, by stimulating increased collagen production and elasticity in the skin. This helps dull the appearance of fine lines and wrinkles, while locking-in moisture. The supplement includes Lipowheat, Polypodium Leucotomos, Beta Carotene, Vitamin C, Green Tea Extract and Hyaluronic Acid.

REBONE™

REBONE™ has been specially formulated with vitamins and minerals that are crucial for bone-building and overall bone health. It is critical to build strong, dense bones whilst you are young and keeping them strong and healthy as you age. The nutraceutical contains AlgaeCal (calcium and magnesium obtained from special algae), Zinc Picolinate, Manganese Bisglycinate, Boron Citrate, Copper II Citrate, Vitamin K_2 (menaquinone-7) and Vitamin D_3 (Calciferol).

RESERENE™

RESERENE™ contains essential nutrients, vitamins and herbs that promote tranquility while helping to calm anxiety. Being able to stay calm and maintain a healthy sleep regimen under duress enables our brain and body to recover and rejuvenate. The nutraceutical contains Passion Flower, Inositol, Lemon Balm and L-Theanine and taken together with the core anti-aging supplements RESPARK™ and REKINDLE™, RESERENE™ promotes healthy aging.

RELINE™

RELINE™ is a supplement that promotes gut and intestine health, by supporting a healthy gastric lining, calming indigestion and discouraging the formation of ulcers. It contains Zinc L-Carnosine, Marshmallow Root, Slippery Elm, Mastic Gum Powder and Gastro Enzyme Blend.

B. The following anti-aging tests are indicated in addition to routine tests:

PHYSICAL EXAM

TEST	RESULT
BMI (the ratio between height and weight)	Between 19.5–25
Waist circumference	Males: 102cm/ 40 inches Females: 88cm/ 35 inches
Hand grip strength	Optimal score according to age tables (This is a good measure of your overall muscle strength and if low, must be improved)
Sit ups in 1 minute — measures abdominal muscle strength	Optimal number according to age table
Push ups in 1 minute — measures upper body and shoulder strength	Optimal number according to age table
Resting pulse	70 or below
Urine PH	Ideal 7.35. If less, indicates increased acidity

LIPID PROFILE

This is an advanced lipid profile which includes LDL particle size and number and HDL particle size and number.

TEST	RESULT
LDL Particles	< 900
Dense LDL particles	< 300
HDL	Males: > 40 Females: > 50
HDL particles	>7,000
Buoyant HDL	Type 2b>1,500
Triglycerides	<150 mg/dl
Triglyceride / HDL ratio	< 2

INFLAMMATORY MARKERS

TEST	RESULT
CRP hs inflammatory marker	<0.9
TNF alpha	<6
Ferritin	40-0 NG/ML
Celiac antibodies to rule out celiac disease	Negative

VASCULAR INFLAMMATION AND BIOMARKERS

TEST	RESULT
Homocysteine — risk factor for vascular disease	<7
Lipoprotein (a)	<5
Apolipoprotein	A1>115
CRP hs	< 3 mg/L

PRE-DIABETES BIOMARKERS

TEST	RESULT
Fasting glucose	80–85 mg/dl
Fasting insulin	<4.5
HBA1c	<5.5
Omega 6/ Omega 3 ratio	0.5–3
Urine microalbumin	0

HORMONES

TEST	RESULT
If stress and adrenal fatigue is suspected, do salivary cortisol test	4 times during 24 hour period and salivary DHEA

Thyroid TSH	**1–2**
Free T3	**3.2–4.2 PG/ML**
Reverse T3	**10–24 NG/DL**
Free T4	**1.3–1.8 NG/ML**
Thyroid antibodies	**0**
Thyroid antibodies — TPO	**0–35 IU/ML**
Females — perimenopausal	**Estrogen and progesterone on 21st day of cycle**
Males — testosterone	**500–1000 NG/DL**
Free testosterone	**6.5–156.5–15 NG/ML**

MINERALS

TEST	**RESULT**
Copper	**90–110 MG/DL**
Zinc	**90–110 MG/DL**
Copper / Zinc ratio	**1**
Selenium	**110–150 NG/ML**
Potassium	**4.5–5.5 meq/L**
Calcium	**8.5–10.5 MG/DL**

Magnesium (best in RBC)	5.2–6.5 MG/DL

TOXINS

TOXIN	RESULTS
Mercury	<5
Lead	<2
Arsenic	<7
Cadmium	<2.5

VITAMIN LEVELS

VITAMIN	RESULTS
Vitamin D	50–80 IU
Vitamin B12	500–1500 PG/ML
Folic Acid	10–25 nmoles/L

OTHER TESTS

Test for arterial health	Non invasive tests to see the status of the blood vessels
Carotid intimal medial thickness	Good method of detecting atherosclerosis
Endopath test	Checks the elasticity of the arteries and the endothelial

	health
Heart rate variability	Assesses the sympathetic nervous system tone of the heart. The higher the stress levels, the more the sympathetic nervous system influences the heart and the higher the risk for heart attack or dangerous arrhythmias

TOP 10 ANTI AGING INTERVENTIONS

1. Hearing test (treat hearing impairment)
2. Exercise —improve fitness
3. Nutrition — eat healthy
4. Stress management
5. Adequate Sleep
6. Purpose and life satisfaction
7. Curcumin
8. Vitamin K3
9. Vitamin D
10. Hormone balance

GLOSSARY

Adrenal fatigue – Stress-related condition that results in extreme exhaustion and a weakened immune system

Aromatase reaction – An enzyme responsible for the biosynthesis of estrogens

Arrhythmias – Heart beats with an irregular or abnormal rhythm

Alzheimer's disease – Progressive mental deterioration that can occur in middle to old age due to the degeneration of the brain

Autonomic nervous system – Consists of the sympathetic and parasympathetic nervous systems

Benign prostatic hyperplasia (BPH) - Enlargement of the prostate gland

Chromosomes – Known as our genes, found in our living cells and carries genetic information

DNA - Double helix molecule that contains the genetic instructions for the functioning, development and reproduction of all living organisms

Endorphins – Hormones secreted by the brain and nervous system to produce physiological functions

Endothelium – A single layer of cells forming the inner layer of blood vessels

Endometrium – Inner lining of the uterus

Epithelial lining – Lining of the bowels

Free radicals - An uncharged molecule that has an unpaired electron

Gait pattern - The way people walk and balance

Glioblastoma - Aggressive brain tumor

Heart rate variability (HRV) - Variation in your heart beat within a specific timeframe

Hypothalamic pituitary axis (HPA) - Regulates cortisol levels

Islet cells - Cells in the pancreas that produce hormones

Macrophages – Large white bloods cells that ingest foreign particles and infectious microorganisms

Metabolic syndrome – A group of medical conditions found simultaneously in a patient, including high blood pressure, excess abdominal fat, high triglycerides

Metabolism – Chemical processes in the body, especially those related to the conversion of food for energy and growth

Microbiota – An ecological community of symbiotic microorganisms consisting of bacteria, fungi and viruses

Mitochondria – An organelle found in large numbers in most cells that facilitates energy production

NAD - Coenzyme that is found in cells and is involved in energy production

Neurotransmitters - A chemical substance that transmits nerve impulses to another nerve or gland

Osteoblasts - A cell that secretes the matrix for bone formation

Osteoporosis – Disorder that causes brittle and fragile bones from loss of calcium and minerals

Parasympathetic nervous system – Known as the rest-and-digest system, it stimulates digestion and slows the heart rate

Perimenopause – Time in a woman's life before menopause begins

Proteinuria – Abnormal quantities of protein in the urine that can damage the kidneys

Sarcopenia – Loss of muscle tissue as a natural part of aging

Senescence – Growing old, aging

Sympathetic nervous system – Activates the fight-or-flight response

Telomere – The segment of DNA that occurs at the end of chromosomes

Telomerase – An enzyme that causes telomeres to lengthen

Vagus nerve – The 10th cranial nerve coming from the brain to the body and supplying the heart, lungs and other organs